# Atlas of Muscle Innervation Zones

Marco Barbero • Roberto Merletti •
Alberto Rainoldi

# Atlas of Muscle Innervation Zones

## Understanding Surface Electromyography and Its Applications

Foreword by Gwendolen Jull

Springer

**Marco Barbero**
Department of Health Sciences
University of Applied Sciences
and Arts of Southern Switzerland,
SUPSI
Manno, Switzerland
e-mail: marco.barbero@supsi.ch

**Roberto Merletti**
LISiN
Department of Electronics
Politecnico di Torino
Turin, Italy
e-mail: roberto.merletti@polito.it

**Alberto Rainoldi**
School of Exercise and Sport
Sciences, SUISM
University of Turin
Italy
e-mail: alberto.rainoldi@unito.it

Additional material to this book can be downloaded from http://extras.springer.com

ISBN 978-88-470-2462-5 ISBN 978-88-470-2463-2 (eBook)

DOI 10.1007/978-88-470-2463-2

Springer Milan Dordrecht Heidelberg London New York
Library of Congress Control Number: 2012938373



**Cover image:** The cover image shows the generation, propagation and extinction of a motor unit action potential as detected on the surface of the skin by a two-dimensional electrode array placed above the biceps brachii muscle. The signal is spatially filtered with a longitudinal double differential filter, along the fiber direction. The interelectrode distance, in the row and column (fiber) direction, is 8 mm and the time interval between each instantaneous image and the next is 2 ms. The images are interpolated to obtain a smooth representation of the potential distributions (see also Fig. 4.5 on page 44).

9 8 7 6 5 4 3 2 1 2012 2013 2014 2015

*Cover design:* Ikona S.r.l., Milan, Italy

Typesetting: Ikona S.r.l., Milan, Italy

Springer-Verlag Italia S.r.l., Via Decembrio 28, I-20137 Milan
Springer is a part of Springer Science+Business Media (www.springer.com)

# Foreword

Research-informed practices are essential for accurate and reliable outcomes in any medical or technical field. Yet there is often a gap between what is known and available in the research arena and what is applied in the field. Translation of the knowledge and information gained from research into practice is a challenge, but one that must be overcome.

The field of electromyography (EMG) is representative of the quite rapid developments that have recently occurred in basic-science knowledge and in technology. A wealth of information has been produced and it has advanced our understanding of the applications and measures of EMG. However, the use of EMG in the applied fields does not always reflect the appropriate dissemination and application of this contemporary knowledge. This means that, in some instances, both the accuracy and the interpretation of the data produced may be questionable. It is for these reasons that the *Atlas of muscle innervation zones: Understanding surface electromyography and its applications* is welcome. Barbero, Merletti, and Rainoldi are highly regarded scientists in the EMG field and they are to be congratulated in their endeavours to improve our understanding of surface EMG and its applications, as authors of a book that both applied scientists and clinicians in the field will appreciate.

They clearly state the purpose of this volume, which is to explain the nature and mechanisms of both EMG generation and the two-dimensional distribution of the potential generated on the skin by the underlying muscles. Their stated aim is to increase the reader's understanding of sEMG rather than to provide recipe-style directives for its applications. Importantly, they also clearly point out the limitations of sEMG, so that pitfalls in the collection or interpretation of signals can be avoided.

This aim has certainly been achieved. The text provides a comprehensive overview of many of the fundamental aspects related to the detection, processing, and interpretation of electrical signals. The authors systematically approach sEMG, from the biological sources of electrical fields and action potentials, to the methods for their detection, and to the physiology of the basic components of sEMG signals. Methods of sEMG signal analysis are discussed. The reader gains a good understanding of the different signals generated by fusiform and pennate muscles. Also highlighted is the importance and relevance of the location of innervations zones for electrode placement over fusiform muscles and the necessity to avoid pitfalls in electrode placement.

The reader is additionally introduced to the concept of mapping of both sEMG signals and EMG variables.

An excellent summary of the key points in the application of sEMG, including under dynamic conditions, is provided. Cognizant of their targeted readership of applied researchers and clinicians, the authors provide examples of applications in the fields of ergonomics, exercise and sports, and surgical workup, all of which bring to life the principles discussed in the text.

The second part of the text consists of an atlas that identifies the innervation zones of 43 muscles accessible to sEMG. This is indeed an invaluable contemporary resource for all those who use sEMG, and the rigour in its construction is evident.

A challenge in writing a book such as this one is to present material that is quite technical in nature in a format that can be understood by the intended readership, which in this case comprises clinicians and applied researchers without a sophisticated background in physics and mathematics. The authors have largely overcome this difficulty by using simple and excellent analogies to illustrate many of the technical aspects. This, in addition to the excellent illustrations that accompany each chapter, gently guides the reader to a good appreciation of sEMG. This book is a valuable resource that will enhance the application and interpretation of sEMG in future field and clinical studies.

Gwendolen Jull
Professor of Physiotherapy
The University of Queensland, Australia

# Preface

Most books on surface electromyography (sEMG) deal with nerve conduction studies, movement analysis (mostly gait), biofeedback, or other clinical applications. They describe the traditional technique, based on one electrode pair, in which a single time-changing signal is detected in one location on the skin. On the other hand, doctoral or post-doctoral researchers with a solid engineering background can avail themselves of the non-clinical "Electromyography: Physiology, Engineering, and Non-Invasive Applications" (IEEE Press Series on Biomedical Engineering), which addresses the issue of EMG detection, processing, and interpretation from the physical and signal-processing points of view.

Our objective is to fill the gap between these two educational approaches while describing new technologies and the physiological information that they extract from sEMG. This information is collected by means of linear or two-dimensional (2D) arrays that provide space-time images of the instantaneous potential distribution as well as maps of sEMG features on the skin below the array. Although this approach has been described in dozens of reports published in scientific journals, it has yet to be adopted in clinical research laboratories.

Perhaps one of the most important topics discussed in this book is the location of the innervation zone(s) in fusiform muscles with fibers parallel to the skin and the related problem of the proper location of a single electrode pair. Since electrode arrays and multichannel amplifiers are not yet commercially available, the technique based on a single electrode pair will continue to be used in the near future, before it is eventually replaced by the more advanced and much more powerful 2D approach. The issue of proper electrode placement will therefore persist for some time.

The purpose of this book is twofold: a) to offer a solid basis of knowledge regarding the mechanisms of sEMG generation and the information that can be extracted from this signal (Part I), and b) to include an Atlas describing the proper electrode positions when a single electrode pair is used (Part II). These two issues are introduced in great detail in Chapter 1. The basic physical concepts concerning fields and potential distributions generated by point sources moving under the skin along the muscle fibers are reviewed in Chapter 2. The physical and physiological phenomena underlying the generation, propagation, and extinction of single-fiber and motor-unit action potentials are described in Chapter 3. The geometry and anatomy of the electrode-muscle system (the sEMG imaging technique) is outlined in Chapter 4. The features of the single-channel sEMG signal and of a 2D representation by multichannel sEMG imaging (amplitude and spectral features, fatigue indexes, and muscle fiber conduction velocity) are described in Chapters 5 and 6. A sample list of applications of sEMG imaging under dynamic conditions and with respect to ergonomics, sports, and obstetrics is provided in Chapter 7.

Part II is an Atlas of the location of the innervation zones of 43 superficial muscles as observed in a sample population of 20 male and 20 female subjects. It provides information on the dispersion of these zones, which are a key anatomical reference that can be identified only by electrophysiological testing. Emphasis is placed on the importance of not locating a single electrode pair in a position that is most likely over or near the innervation zone of the muscle. The failure to take this precaution has been the source of considerable confusion in the scientific literature (and possibly in the clinical findings) related to sEMG. It is our hope that the information provided in the Atlas will greatly improve the knowledge and abilities of students, researchers and practitioners in the fields of physical therapy, movement sciences, ergonomics, sport medicine, space medicine, and obstetrics.

Three areas of knowledge are merged in this work and they reflect the training and professional experience of the authors. Specific expertise in clinical physiotherapy was provided by Marco Barbero. Extensive experience in the research and teaching of biomedical and rehabilitation engineering was provided by Roberto Merletti. Specific competence in physics, movement analysis, and movement and sport sciences was contributed by Alberto Rainoldi. We hope that our collaboration will be helpful to students and practitioners in integrating the body of knowledge provided by academic courses, most of which, unfortunately, do not yet include material concerning the rapidly growing field of sEMG.

We are indebted to Gwendolen Jull (Professor of Physiotherapy at The University of Queensland, Australia) for the foreword to this book, and to the many collaborators and students who made this book possible by contributing to the collection and presentation of the data with their enthusiastic and careful work.

May 2012

Marco Barbero
Roberto Merletti
Alberto Rainoldi

# Acknowledgments

The results presented in this book summarize many years of work carried out by students and researchers. Their efforts would not have been possible without the support of grants provided to the University of Applied Sciences and Arts of Southern Switzerland (SUPSI) by Thim van der Laan Foundation, to the Laboratory for Engineering of the Neuromuscular System (LISiN, Politecnico di Torino) by the European Commission, the Regional Administration of Piemonte, Compagnia di San Paolo and Fondazione CRT, and to the School of Exercise and Sport Sciences (SUISM, University of Turin) by the Compagnia di San Paolo and Fondazione ISEF.
The authors would like to thank these institutions as well as the individuals listed below.

The following individuals contributed to the data collection as well as the processing and organization of the material:

**Roberto Bergamo** Lab. for Engineering of the Neuromuscular System, Politecnico di Torino, Turin, Italy

**Matteo Beretta Piccoli** Department of Health Sciences, University of Applied Sciences and Arts of Southern Switzerland (SUPSI), Manno, Switzerland

**Gennaro Boccia** School of Exercise and Sport Sciences (SUISM), University of Turin, Italy

**Carolin Heitz** Department of Health Sciences, University of Applied Sciences and Arts of Southern Switzerland (SUPSI), Landquart, Switzerland

**Andrea Merlo** Lab. for Engineering of the Neuromuscular System, Politecnico di Torino, Turin, Italy

**Lorenzo Nannucci** Lab. for Engineering of the Neuromuscular System, Politecnico di Torino, Turin, Italy

**Michel Rozzi** Department of Health Sciences, University of Applied Sciences and Arts of Southern Switzerland (SUPSI), Manno, Switzerland

**Costantino Sanfilippo** Lab. for Engineering of the Neuromuscular System, Politecnico di Torino, Turin, Italy

**Carlo Spirolazzi** School of Physiotherapy, Vita-Salute University San Raffaele, Milan, Italy

**Massimiliano Titolo** Lab. for Engineering of the Neuromuscular System, Politecnico di Torino, Turin, Italy

**Enrico Tomasoni** School of Exercise and Sport Sciences (SUISM), University of Turin, Italy

**Marianne Wüthrich** Department of Health Sciences, University of Applied Sciences and Arts of Southern Switzerland (SUPSI), Landquart, Switzerland

The following individuals contributed material and critical revision of the text by providing advice and suggestions:

**Deborah Falla** Pain Clinic, Center for Anesthesiology, University Hospital Göttingen, Germany

**Alessio Gallina** Lab. for Engineering of the Neuromuscular System, Politecnico di Torino, Turin, Italy

**Roberto Gatti** Università Vita e Salute, S. Raffaele Hospital, Milan, Italy

**Taian Vieira** Lab. for Engineering of the Neuromuscular System, Politecnico di Torino, Turin, Italy

We are indebted to all of them for their dedication and professionalism in contributing their time and expertise to the completion of this book.

Thanks are extended also to the SUPSI Laboratory of Visual Culture for collaboration in the preparation of effective anatomical illustrations.

# Contents

**Part I**

# Abbreviations

| | |
|---|---|
| 1D | one dimensional |
| 2D | two-dimensional |
| ALF | anatomical landmark frame |
| AP | action potential |
| ARV | average rectified value |
| CV | muscle fiber conduction velocity |
| EAS | external anal sphincter muscle |
| ECG | electrocardiogram or electrocardiography |
| EEG | electroencephalogram or electroencephalography |
| EMG | electromyogram or electromyography |
| IED | inter-electrode distance |
| IZ | innervation zone |
| LSD, LDD | longitudinal single differential, longitudinal double differential |
| MAV | mean average value |
| MNF, MDF | mean spectral frequency, median spectral frequency |
| MRV | mean rectified value |
| MSV | mean square value |
| MU | motor unit |
| MUAP | motor unit action potential |
| MVC | maximal voluntary contraction |
| NMJ | neuromuscular junction |
| RMS | root mean square |
| sEMG | surface electromyogram or electromyography |
| TSD, TDD | transversal single differential, transversal double differential |

# Part I

*Roberto Merletti*

# Introduction and Applications of Surface EMG

1

**Abstract**

Despite technical progress and the many applications of surface electromyography (sEMG) reported in the literature, its use remains limited, mostly because of insufficient technology transfer and educational efforts. This book is aimed at physical therapists, movement scientists, ergonomists, and other health professionals and its purpose is to provide them with information on the correct use, but also on the many forms of misuse, of sEMG. Although it has no clinical objectives and it is not a clinical manual, this book nonetheless includes several applications, which are listed in this chapter and expanded upon in Chapter 7.

## 1.1 Objectives

In the last two decades, the technologies for detecting, processing, and interpreting bioelectrical signals have improved tremendously. This is particularly true for surface electromyography (sEMG), the study of signals generated by skeletal muscles and detected on the skin. Regrettably, despite the hundreds of scientific publications and the many engineering congresses and academic courses on the bioelectrical signal processing techniques applicable to sEMG, the medical and health professions have benefitted very little from this explosion of knowledge, mostly because of the paucity of training, courses, seminars, and workshops aimed at their members.

This book was written to fill this gap and is therefore intended for physical therapists, experts in movement sciences, ergonomists, and other professionals in related fields. It focuses on the detection and interpretation of sEMG, touching only briefly on clinical applications. Rather, the primary purpose of the material contained herein is to translate the new knowledge in the field of sEMG—which is strongly based on mathematics and physics and accordingly structured in equations and algorithms—into a number of concepts, examples, and didactic figures that can be readily applied while at the same time providing guidelines for health professionals.

Thus, this book does *not* offer directions, recipes, or instructions on equipment usage or on sEMG-based diagnosis or treatments. Nor does it discuss workplace design, worker monitoring, or the prevention of surgical lesions to the neuromuscular system (such as episiotomy). Instead, it seeks to *inform* potential sEMG users about the state of the art and the technological developments that can be expected in the near future. It has been left up to the reader to investigate the hundreds of applications, to develop clinical research objectives, and perhaps even to write a second volume, one that covers these topics. Some of the devices and methods described in this book are prototypes that have been tested successfully in research labs and in selected clinical environments. They are ready to be the subjects of academic courses, and their widespread clinical use by competent and trained operators is encouraged.

It is our hope that this book will provide a solid support for medical and health professionals. In

M. Barbero, R. Merletti, A. Rainoldi, *Atlas of Muscle Innervation Zones*,

Part II, the guidelines on the location of the innervation zones of 47 superficial muscles, and therefore on the proper location of a single electrode pair, will no doubt be of particular interest.

Muscles are the motors that allow us to move, and the mechanisms of operation of these motors constitute a masterpiece of engineering. Unscrambling these mechanisms and cracking the code by which the motors are controlled are major challenges, and much remains to be learned. Applications of the available information and insights into the murkier areas of the muscular system demand thorough knowledge of the signal-generation mechanisms. Such knowledge is essential, both at the research level, for a deeper understanding of the neuromuscular system, and at the clinical level, for the purpose of detecting fatigue, understanding the control strategies and physiological mechanisms altered by aging, recognizing the effects of the lack of exercise and those of sport training, as well as elucidating disease mechanisms.

Too many health operators draw conclusions based on the use of a single-channel EMG signal or make clinical decisions without being completely aware of what kind of information this signal *can* provide (in terms of anatomy, physiology, biophysics, and pathology) or *not* provide. Moreover, the information obtained from the single-channel signal is incomplete and sometimes misleading, like a voice through a noisy phone line, leaving it open to interpretation in more than one way, depending on the modality of signal detection and processing. However, it must be borne in mind that the information content of the signal is limited and we cannot extract more information than it actually contains. Health operators must therefore be familiar with these modalities and aware of their potential, but also of their limitations and possible misinterpretations.

## 1.2 Two Simple Examples from Related Fields

Example 1. Suppose that a movie is projected onto a screen but the screen is covered by a black canvas with two holes. Only two spots of the screen are visible. Can we figure out what the movie is about? Can we extrapolate the information contained in the images that are evolving in time? What kind of information can we reasonably expect to obtain from this strongly limited view? This situation is similar to the one in which we have a continuously changing and complex potential distribution on the skin (that we cannot see) and we place only one pair of sensors to detect a single time-changing potential difference. This type of situation is described in Sect. 2.1.

Example 2. We apply microphones to the external side of a wall of a room where many people are talking or an orchestra is playing. Of course we detect sounds. Do they allow us to distinguish the instruments or understand the simultaneous conversations taking place in the room? Are there preferred positions for the microphones? Would increasing the number of microphones help in distinguishing the instruments or in understanding the voices and conversations? Could we "focus" the microphones or process the detected sounds in such a way so as to isolate at least some of the instruments or conversations? Would our understanding be furthered by introducing and moving a few microphones into the room? How many microphones would we need? Would it help to cover the wall with a grid of microphones? Could the signals from the microphones be processed in such a way so as to "focus" our detection system on a particular region of space, thus allowing the detection of at least the conversations going on (or the instruments located) in that region? This situation, also described in Sect. 2.1, is similar to one in which the sources are electric-field generators.

In some cases, detecting, processing, and understanding sEMG signals is analogous to understanding a movie through a few holes made in a canvas covering the screen, or understanding conversations through a few microphones placed on the outside (or even the inside!) of the wall of a room. Some information can be recovered, some cannot. Being aware of this fact and making the best use of the available information, without misinterpreting it and, above all, without interpreting the missing information, are of paramount importance in current sEMG techniques. This is the reason why operators must be aware of sEMG's limitations and why they must be trained to properly understand both the nature and significance of the available signals and the available blurred information. Providing this training, together with insight into the limitations of the technique, is the main purpose of this book.

The sEMG signal offers a window on the motor (the muscle) as well as on its controller (the nervous system). This window is small and what we can see behind it is often distorted by the curved and not fully transparent glass of the window itself. If this book induces in its readers a sense of marvel and curiosity, a feeling of respect toward the beauty and elegance of the sEMG system's design, a desire to understand it by breaking its codes and unraveling its rules, and the motivation to address the challenges that are still open, and therefore to pursue some of the many research tasks, then our goal will be completely fulfilled. But even if it simply makes the reader aware of the possibilities, limitations, current misinterpretations, and future potential breakthroughs of sEMG techniques, so that mistakes are prevented by the increased knowledge, then we, as its authors, have achieved a major success.

## 1.3 Applications of sEMG

Whether we record it or not, a distribution of electric potential is present on the skin surface. This distribution contains information related to the sources of the electric field that generate it, i.e., the action potentials (AP) propagating along the muscle fibers that make up the muscle. These sources are described in Chapter 3 but at this point we can imagine them as tiny batteries, between the two poles of which an electric field is generated, in the surrounding space. Every one of these fields contributes to the potential differences between any two points chosen on the skin. This potential difference is the sum of the contributions made by the many sources present in the muscle and those resulting from noise and interferences. The modality of signal detection and processing depends on the questions being asked and the reasons for collecting the sEMG signal. In some cases, two (correctly placed) electrodes may be sufficient; in other cases dozens of electrodes may be required.

Consider again the two examples given in Sect. 1.2. Some of the very simple questions that we can ask are: Is a movie being projected on the screen, or not? Are people talking in the room on the other side of the wall, or not? Quite obviously, a few sensors, like the holes in the canvas covering the screen or the microphones applied to the wall, may be sufficient to answer questions of this type. Similarly, only a very few electrodes applied on the skin covering a muscle may allow us to determine whether the muscle is generating any signal, or not.

There are also questions of intermediate complexity: Are the voices in the room getting louder? Do they change pitch? Are certain colors appearing more or less often on the screen? Are the images changing progressively faster or slower? Are the speakers increasing or decreasing in number? Are they having conversations or singing in unison in a choir? These questions also have their equivalent in sEMG. Is the signal getting stronger? Is it changing pitch? Is its intensity different in different regions of the skin? Do these features change with time or aging or diseases? Are the sources increasing or decreasing in number? Are they somehow synchronized or changing in unison or repeating a pattern? Much more complex questions (most of which are still unanswered today) concern the movie itself, the subject of the conversations going on across the wall, etc.

Most of the current sEMG applications are limited to answering questions of the very simple type indicated above. A few applications attempt to answer questions of intermediate difficulty. Very few research labs and even fewer clinical institutions address the most difficult questions and no clinical applications are based, at this time, on the (yet quite controversial and incomplete) answers to them.

Despite the need for more research concerning the most difficult (but physiologically most relevant) issues, the current level of technology provides information useful in many different fields, as described in Chapter 7. Some of these fields are briefly described in Table 1.1.

**Table 1.1** Some fields and areas of current applications of surface EMG

| Field | Surface EMG Applications |
|---|---|
| *Neurophysiological and medical research* | Functional neurology, investigation of spasticity, cramps, and related phenomena<br>Orthopedics and neuromuscular surgery<br>Gait and posture analysis<br>Aging |
| *Rehabilitation* | Neurological rehabilitation and neurorehabilitation engineering<br>Physical therapy and active training therapy<br>Assessment of treatment effectiveness, monitoring of a patient's improvement<br>Use of EMG from residual muscles for the external control of paralyzed human extremities or of a prosthesis<br>Biofeedback applications |
| *Ergonomics* | Analysis and ergonomic design of workplaces<br>Risk prevention and early detection of disorder development by periodic monitoring |
| *Sports and movement science* | Biomechanics and movement analysis<br>Monitoring the effectiveness of strength or endurance training<br>Sport injury rehabilitation<br>Optimal design of sports equipment or instruments |
| *Others* | Assessment of neuromuscular deterioration in space missions in microgravity conditions<br>Accompanying episiotomy during child delivery to minimize the risk of sphincter denervation<br>Identification of the optimal location for botulinum toxin injection<br>Control of robots and machinery<br>In the performing arts, using sEMG to control music or lights |

# 2 Basic Concepts Concerning Fields and Potential Distributions of Stationary and Moving Point Sources

**Abstract**

This chapter addresses the issue of associating the location and nature of the electric field sources below the surface of a conductive medium with the corresponding potential distribution on that surface. Single-point sources (monopoles), pairs of opposite sources (dipoles), and pairs of dipoles (tripoles or quadrupoles) are investigated together with the detection modalities of the surface potential (monopolar, differential, etc.). The electric potentials generated by sources moving under these detection systems are described using a qualitative approach. The general concept of a spatial filter is introduced.

## 2.1 The Concept of Potential

Bioelectric signals are generated by organs such as the heart (electrocardiogram, ECG) and the brain (electroencephalogram, EEG) as well as by the muscles (electromyogram, EMG) and other structures, e.g., the stomach, gut (electrogastrogram, EGG), and eyes (electro-oculogram, EOG). In all these cases the signals derive from sources of electric fields that are inside the body, at some distance from the skin, where the potentials of these fields can be detected by means of electrodes.

These sources are the action potentials (APs) generated by excitable cells. The nature of these potentials is discussed in Chapter 3. The sources are surrounded by a medium that is more or less electrically conductive, i.e., it enables the flow of electrical charges (ions). An electric field is a force field (like gravity) that can produce the movement of particles (ions move in an electric field like particles in a gravitational field) and can be detected by special sensors (such as accelerometers or inclinometers in the case of a gravitational field). We can imagine other types of fields, such as a light intensity field generated by a light bulb, or a color-intensity field, a sound field, a pressure field, a temperature field, etc.

While some of these fields are immediately perceived by human senses, others are not. For example, we can perceive the different temperatures along a metal bar when one end is heated and the other is not, or the energy accumulated by a raindrop falling from a cloud along the gravitational field of the Earth, or the pressure field (sound) generated by an explosion whose pressure wave diffuses in the surrounding space, or the light field generated by a light spot in the nearby space. On the other hand, we cannot perceive the electric field generated by the two poles of a battery (or by our heart or brain or muscles), the magnetic field generated by the North and South Poles of the Earth or by a magnet, or the field emitted by a radio station.

However, we can perceive the effects of some of these fields, even if we do not "see" them. If we touch the two poles of a high-voltage battery or an outlet of the power line we get an "electric shock". We can see the needle of a compass align with a magnetic field that we do not perceive. We perceive the effect of a small stone dropped from a distance of one meter above our hand and falling along the

M. Barbero, R. Merletti, A. Rainoldi, *Atlas of Muscle Innervation Zones*,

gravitational field of the Earth. The same stone, falling along the same gravitational field, but from the top of a building, has a very different effect on our hand because of the energy it has accumulated moving along the gravitational field. This "potential energy," accumulated by particles "potentially" moving along a field, is always referred to two points. It should be noted that the potential exists even if we do not "test" it. The stone suspended at the top of a building has a potential even if it not released, the hot metal bar has a potential even if we do not touch it, and a light bulb generates a potential even if we are blind and cannot see it. Thus, we can have a temperature potential between two points of a bar with one end heated, a gravitational potential between two different heights, A and B, one higher than the other, or an electric potential between two points within a conducting medium (such as a biological tissue) to which the poles of an electric generator are applied (not necessarily to the same points we are observing).

Electric generators within our body generate electric fields and (with the proper instruments) we can measure potential differences between the points we have access to, that is, on the skin. It is unfortunate that our senses cannot "see" electric field distributions or electric potentials between pairs of points on the skin. If we could see electric fields and potentials as colors (just as we see fields of electromagnetic radiation in the wavelength range of 0.4 μm to 0.8 μm as colors from violet to red) we would have a totally different perception of the activities of our body, based on the colors appearing on our skin. This ability would allow us to see waves of colors rapidly moving and continuously changing on our skin in a symphony of differently colored moving clouds reflecting the activity of our heart, brain, and muscles (see Chapter 6).

An important area of electrophysiology investigates the way these potentials appear and evolve on the skin, giving us a crude hint about the fields and potential distributions that we cannot perceive with our senses because we do not have the appropriate sensory organs (some animals, like sharks, can detect the electric fields generated by their prey). The purpose of these electrophysiological studies is to identify the features and mechanisms of the correctly or incorrectly operating organs that are generating those fields and potentials. We know the how and why of the P, QRS, and T waves of the ECG of a normal heart and we can use the ECG to investigate the functioning of the heart and its abnormalities. We understand how the EEG is modified just before and during an epileptic crisis and we can use this information to assess these patients. By contrast, much less is known about how the EMG signal reflects the operation of the muscle and of its controller but a considerable amount of information is there, waiting to be extracted. This information will provide insight into the muscle itself as well as into the strategies of its control.

The skin is far from the sources of the electric field generated in the heart, brain, and muscles. In fact, the presence of the skin and of the interposed tissues blurs the fields generated by these sources, just as turbid water blurs a light spot at some depth. It would be desirable to get closer to the body's electric field sources with artificial sensory organs in order to obtain clearer electrical images. This can be done, albeit rather crudely, using invasive techniques. Intracavitary heart catheters can detect the activity of the His bundle, and electrodes placed on the brain's membranes (or needles placed into the brain) can detect localized activities. Muscles can be penetrated with needles and thin wires more easily and with much less risk than the heart or brain. For this reason, needle (invasive) EMG was developed much earlier than surface (non-invasive) EMG and is today widely used to detect myogenic or neurogenic disorders.

## 2.2 Single Stationary Point Source

To better understand the EMG images generated by the muscle fiber APs on the skin surface, we can make use of an optical analogy. As a first step, consider a light bulb at some depth in a moderately transparent medium (e.g., turbid water). The light field generated by the bulb will create a halo on the surface of the water, as indicated in Fig. 2.1a. We can define a coordinate system having two perpendicular axes, x and y, on the surface of the liquid and a vertical axis indicating depth

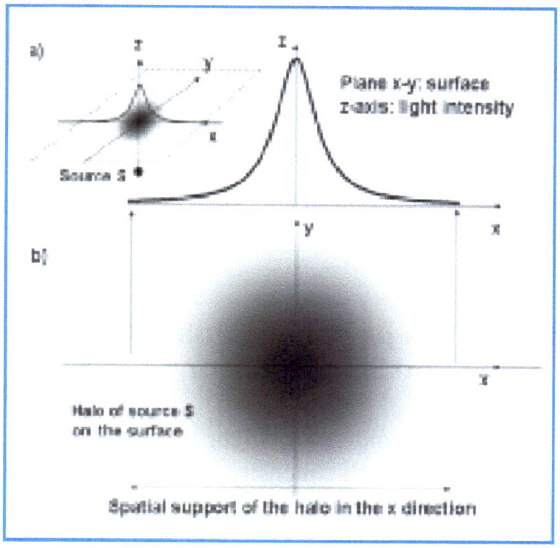


**Fig. 2.1** **a** Image of the potential distribution on the x-y plane generated by a point source S, for example, a light under water. The halo of the light on the surface is shown together with the light intensity in the x-z plane, where the z axis depicts the light intensity. **b** The halo of the light source S represents the brightness of the light (potential) in two dimensions (x-y plane) and the profile of this potential along the x axis. The concept of spatial support of the potential distribution is introduced. Due to the circular symmetry, the profile depicted in the x-z plane is the same in any other plane incorporating the z axis. In a non-isotropic medium, the halo would not be circular (e.g., it might be elliptical)

(below the surface) or light intensity (above the surface), referred to as the z direction. We can also imagine the light halo on the surface (the x-y plane in Fig. 2.1b). This halo represents the light intensity of any point on the x-y plane above the bulb with respect to a distant point. The intensity is inversely proportional to the distance of the point from the bulb, that is if the distance doubles the intensity becomes half, if the distance triples the intensity becomes one third, and so on. Of course, the point of highest intensity is the one with the shortest distance from the source; that is, the one directly above it. The intensity along the x axis is described in Fig. 2.1b as the region where the bell-like surface, representing the intensity, is not negligible. This curve represents the light (or the electric) monopolar potential generated by source S (of light or an electric field) as measured at every point of the line where the x-y plane intersects the x-z plane with respect to a distant point not affected by this or other sources. If the system has circular symmetry, the curve is the same in all directions.

A step forward is presented in Fig. 2.2, where a few light sensors (A–E) have been placed on the surface of the liquid at distances $R_A$, $R_B$, $R_C$, $R_D$,

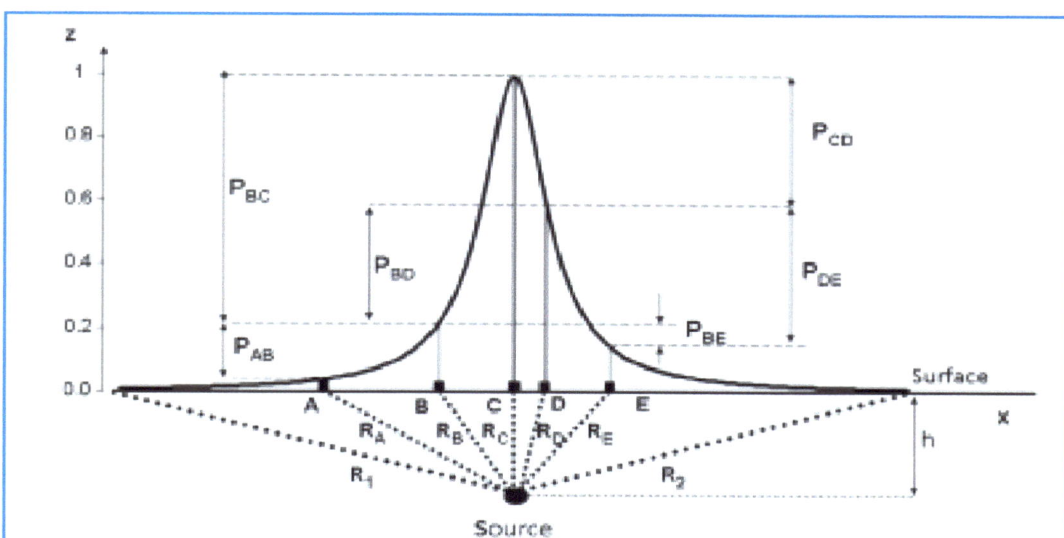


**Fig. 2.2** A potential profile (such as that shown in Fig. 2.1) is sampled by sensors placed at points A, B, C, D, and E on the surface above source S. The potential values are inversely proportional to the distances of the sensors from the source S. These readings are called "monopolar" and are referred to a remote point at zero potential. Potential differences between sensors ($P_{AB}$, $P_{BC}$, $P_{BD}$, etc.) are indicated. These readings are called "differential"

and $R_E$ from the source. The distances $R_1$ and $R_2$ define the spatial "support" of the halo along the x axis; that is, the region beyond which the light is too weak to be detected.

The vertical lines from the sensors indicate the light intensity ("monopolar" potential with respect to a distant spot) under each sensor. The difference between the potentials of any two electrodes ($P_{AB}$, $P_{BC}$, etc.) provides the "differential" reading between those two electrodes. A few considerations are self-evident: it is clear that (a) the point with the highest potential is just above the source; (b) the farther a pair of sensors is from the source, the more similar the two potentials and the smaller their potential difference; (c) the closer two sensors are to each other, the smaller their potential difference; (d) the deeper the source, the lower the potential bell curve; and (e) two sensors at the same distance from the source, on the right and left sides, will detect the same potentials. Figure 2.3 illustrates additional considerations. Two sources, $S_1$ and $S_2$, are placed at depths $h_1$ and $h_2$. The monopolar light potentials detected by sensors A and B, and generated separately by $S_1$ and $S_2$, are indicated together with the differential potentials detected by the same sensors. Sensors C and D, near the edge of the halo, detect similar small monopolar potentials from the two sources (the distance of the sensors from $S_1$ and from $S_2$ is about the same).

## 2.3 Single Moving Point Source and Single Sensor

Consider the underwater light described in Fig. 2.1, its halo, and the intensity (potential) profile it generates on the surface. Suppose now that the light source is moving to the right along a line parallel to the surface and to the x axis with a constant velocity v. Since the halo is generated by the source, it moves with it at the same velocity, along the x axis. Suppose now that we have a point-like light sensor A placed along the x axis on the surface: this sensor is fixed and provides an indication of the light it detects as a function of time.

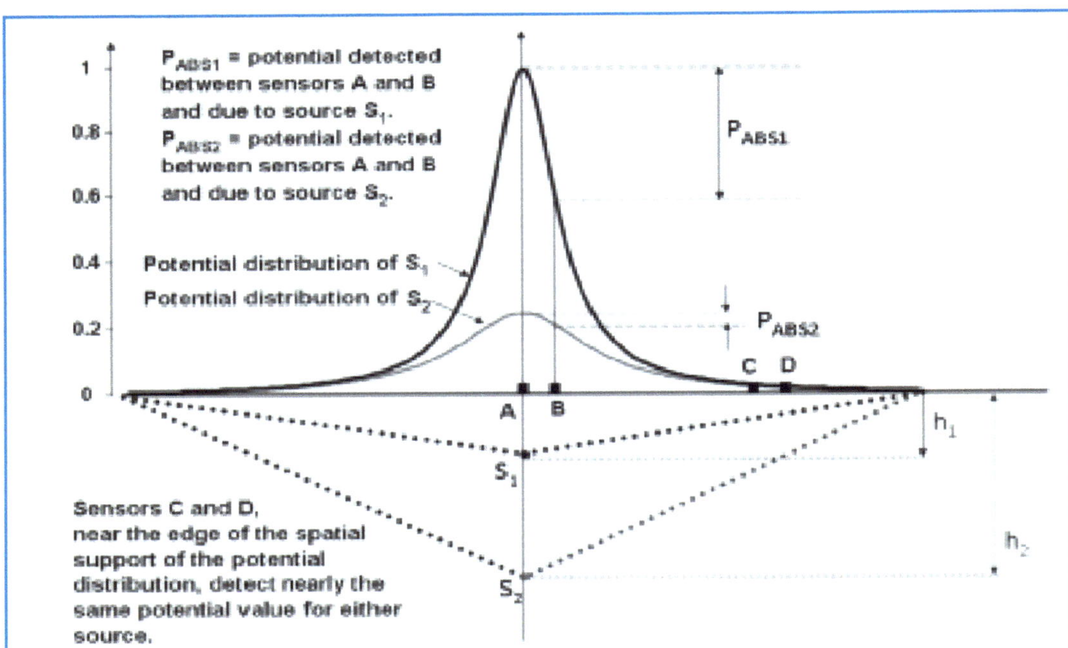


Fig. 2.3 Monopolar potential profiles of two sources, $S_1$ and $S_2$, at different depths $h_1$ and $h_2$, and the potential differences detected between sensor pairs A-B and C-D. Deeper sources generate lower and "smoother" potentials. Differential readings from the same electrode pair are smaller for deeper sources than for more superficial sources

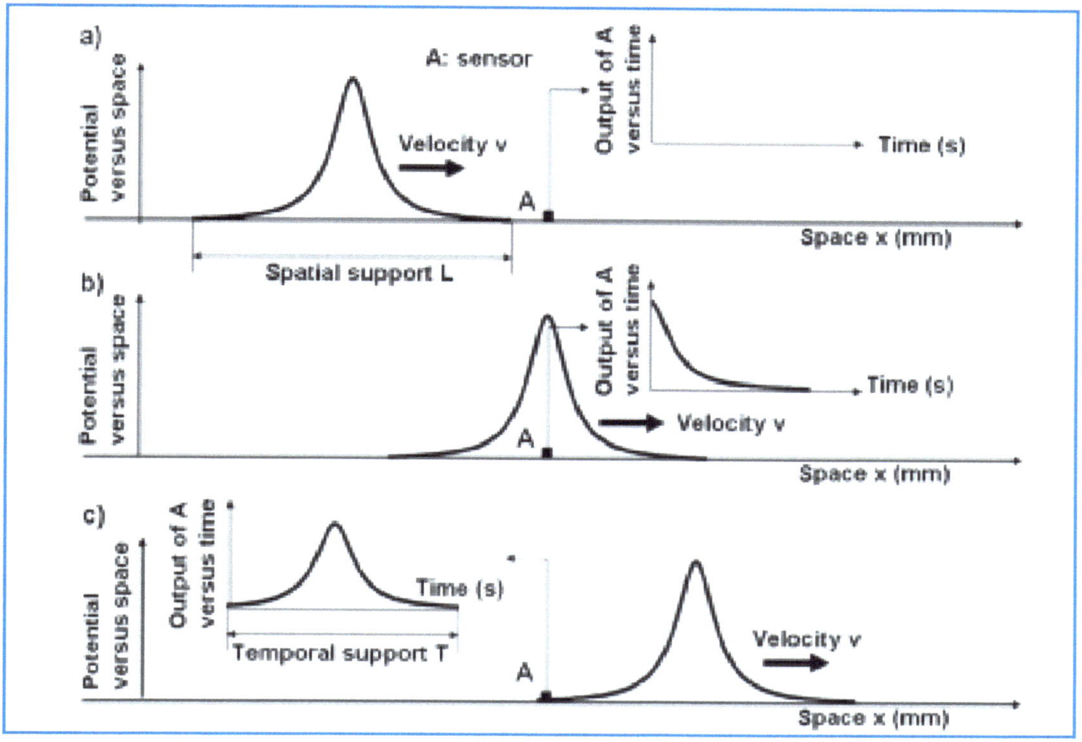


**Fig. 2.4** A potential profile (in space) propagates with velocity v from left to right, under detector A, which reads a potential vs. time. **a** The potential distribution approaches sensor A. **b** The potential is centered below A. **c** The potential profile has moved past A. The spatial support L and the time support T are related by T = L/v because it takes T seconds for the profile to move by L meters

When the entire spatial support of the potential profile is to the left of sensor A, nothing is detected. As the halo (and the potential profile along the x axis) slide under the sensor, the latter provides an output proportional to the light intensity under it. This condition is depicted in Fig. 2.4a.

When the source is exactly below the sensor, the detected potential is maximal and half of the potential profile will have been detected as a function of time. This condition is depicted in Fig. 2.4b.

When the source has moved sufficiently to the right of sensor A, so that the entire profile in space (that is, the entire spatial support of the halo) is to the right of A, the potential detected by sensor A is zero again. This condition is depicted in Fig. 2.4c.

We can see that the shape of the light intensity signal detected by A vs. time is identical to the shape of the light potential profile in space along the x axis, but it may be wider or narrower in time depending on the source velocity.

Let us consider a numerical example. Suppose that the spatial support of the halo along the x axis is 0.020 m (20 mm) and that the source moves with a velocity of 4 m/s (4 mm/ms) underneath the x axis and parallel to it. How long will it take the profile, having a support L = 20 mm, to pass completely under the sensor? Every ms, the source and its potential profile move in space by 4 mm and therefore take L/v (20 mm/4 mm/s) ms. Therefore, after 5 ms the profile will have moved entirely to the right of sensor A and the time duration of the detected signal (that is, the time support of the profile) will be 5 ms. As a second example, consider a spatial support of 0.050 m (50 mm) and a velocity of 5 m/s (5 mm/ms): the temporal support T of the signal detected by sensor A will be T = L/v = 0.050 m / 5 m/s = 0.010 s, that is T = L/v = 50 mm/5 mm/ms = 10 ms. The reader is invited to work out other, similar numerical examples.

To further clarify the relationship between

waves of potential in space and time, consider a wave moving in the sea and a boat floating on the sea. As the wave approaches, the boat progressively rises until it is on top of the wave, above sea level. As the wave moves forward the boat gradually falls and, after the wave has passed, the boat is again at sea level. The boat's position (in the x-y plane) does not change but its gravitational potential first increases and then decreases following the shape of the wave. We can describe such a wave as a spatio-temporal phenomenon, since the wave is described in space and its position changes over time, generating a temporal phenomenon, since the boat goes up and down, i.e., along the z axis, in time but its position on the water surface, i.e., in the x-y plane, does not change.

The time needed for the boat to rise and then fall to its original position is given by the ratio between the width of the wave (its spatial support) and the velocity of the wave. Therefore, the same time event can be caused by either a narrow wave (space) moving slowly or a wider wave moving faster. Clearly, the time support of the boat oscillation by itself cannot provide us with information concerning the width of the wave in space or its velocity.

Of course, the same concepts and calculations apply if the source generates an electric field and the detector detects an electric potential rather than a light potential or the height of a boat above resting sea level (gravitational potential). Examples with animations are available on the website www.lisin.polito.it.

## 2.4 Single Moving Point Source and Two Sensors

Consider now the case shown in Fig. 2.5, where two sensors, A and B, are placed on the surface of the medium at a fixed distance d from each other and are aligned with the x axis, along which the field source and its halo move with velocity v. Let us assume that the distance d is smaller than the spatial support L of the potential distribution V along x. Furthermore, consider a device detecting the potentials in A and B and computing their difference. This device is depicted as a triangle in Fig. 2.5 and its output is collected at point C. The potential of point C is therefore $V_C = V_A + (-V_B) = V_A - V_B$; that is, $V_C$ is the sum of $V_A$ and $V_B$, with the latter defined as a negative value $(-V_B)$.

The potential profile moves to the right with constant velocity v and in Fig. 2.5a–c is depicted in three positions: as it approaches sensors A and B, when it is centered between them, and when it has passed them. Each sensor detects a potential profile vs. time, as indicated in Fig. 2.4. In Fig. 2.5d, the profile detected by sensor A is indicated as $V_A$ (dashed line) and the profile detected by sensor B as $-V_B$ (dotted line). The sum of $V_A$ and $-V_B$ is indicated as $V_C$ (solid line).

A few observations are immediately evident from Fig. 2.5. When the potential profile V is far from the sensors (either to their right or their left), both $V_A$ and $V_B$ are zero and their difference $V_C$ is zero. When the potential profile V approaches the sensors from the left (Fig. 2.5a) and begins to slide under them, $V_A$ is greater than $V_B$ ($V_A > V_B$) and $V_C$ is positive ($V_C > 0$).

When the potential profile V is centered between A and B, $V_A$ is equal to $V_B$ ($V_A = V_B$) and the potential of C is zero ($V_C = 0$).

When the potential profile V moves further, $V_A$ becomes smaller than $V_B$ ($V_A < V_B$) and their difference $V_C$ is negative ($V_C < 0$) until the potential is totally to the right of B and we have again $V_A = 0$, $V_B = 0$ and $V_C = 0$. The potential $V_C$ is depicted with a solid line in Fig. 2.5d, which shows a positive phase and a negative phase. The delay between the peaks of $V_A$ and $V_B$ in time is t and it is equal to the time it takes for the peak of V to move from A to B. This time is the distance between A and B divided by the velocity of V, that is $t = d/v$.

This example illustrates a concept that is of fundamental importance in understanding the differential surface EMG: that a potential distribution moving in space and detected by one or more sensors generates potentials that evolve in time.

## 2.5 A Sinusoidal Wave Moving in Space Under Two Sensors

To further clarify the concept illustrated above, consider the example given in Sect. 2.2, in which the potential V is represented by a wave in the sea and, in

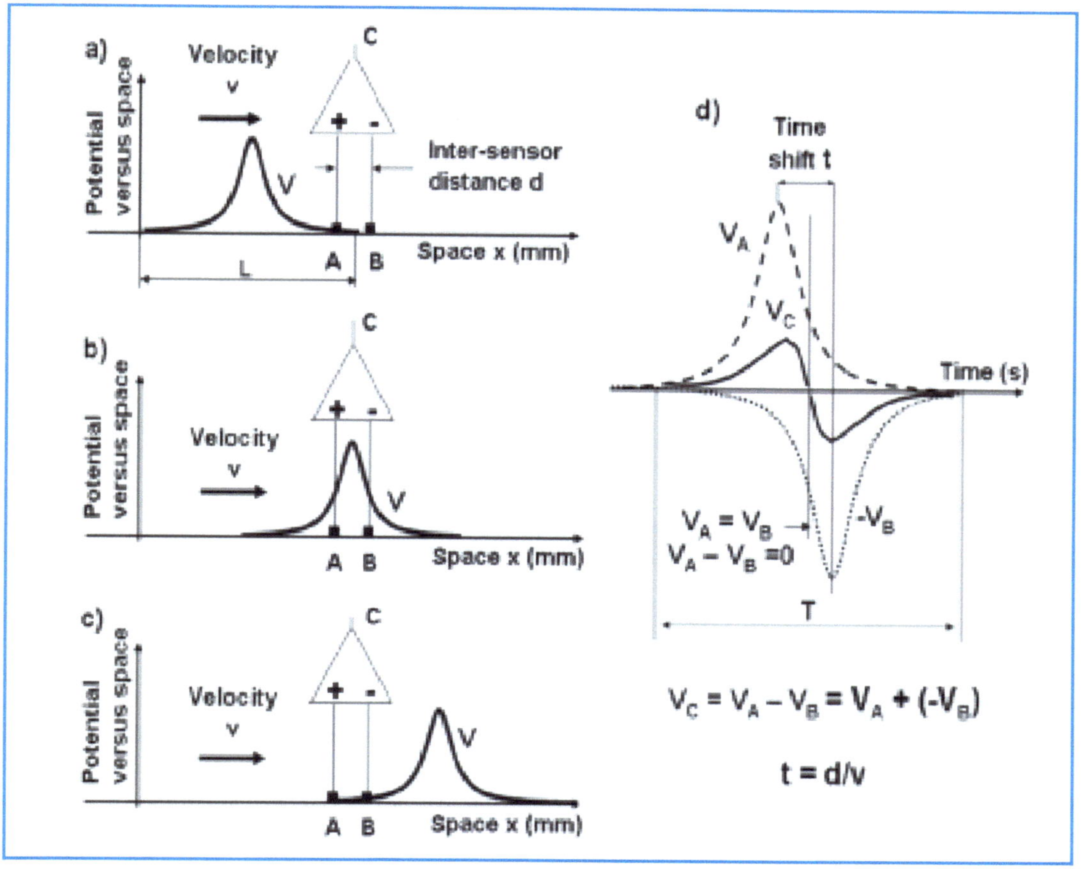


Fig. 2.5 A potential profile V (in space) moves under a pair of sensors A and B, generating two monopolar readings, VA and VB (– VB is shown), and their difference VC. **a** The potential profile V (in space) approaches the sensor pair A-B. **b** The potential profile V is centered under the sensors. **c** The potential profile V has passed the sensors. **d** Monopolar potentials VA and VB detected by sensors A and B and their difference VC

this case, sensors A and B by two floating boats at a fixed distance from each other. The difference in height between the two boats as the wave V passes under them corresponds to the potential measured in C and is described in time by $V_C$. These potentials are detected in A, B, and C and evolve in time. While V describes a potential profile in space, $V_A$, $V_B$, and $V_C$ describe potential profiles in time.

A number of additional considerations are now left to the reader. How are the peak to peak amplitude and the time support T of $V_C$ related to the velocity v, to the inter-sensor distance d, and to the spatial support L? What happens to $V_C$ if the inter-sensor distance d increases such that it either reaches L or is greater than L? What if d is very small with respect to L, such as 5% of L?

The analogy with a wave in the sea and two boats suggests further considerations of the spatio-temporal relationships due to traveling waves. Consider a sequence of identical waves in the sea that, for the sake of simplicity, have a sinusoidal shape (see Sect. 5.3). This example is depicted in Fig. 2.6a, in which the peaks and troughs of the waves sequentially move under A and B at velocity v. The heights of boats A and B (potentials A and B) increase and decrease sinusoidally in time as V moves to the right in space. Actually, the height of B follows that of A with a delay $t = d/v$, that is the time it takes the wave to go from A to B.

Figure 2.6b shows the potentials $V_A$, $V_B$, and $V_C$ as functions of time. Note that $V_B$ is depicted as $V_B$ and not as $-V_B$ and that $V_C = V_A - V_B$ is zero

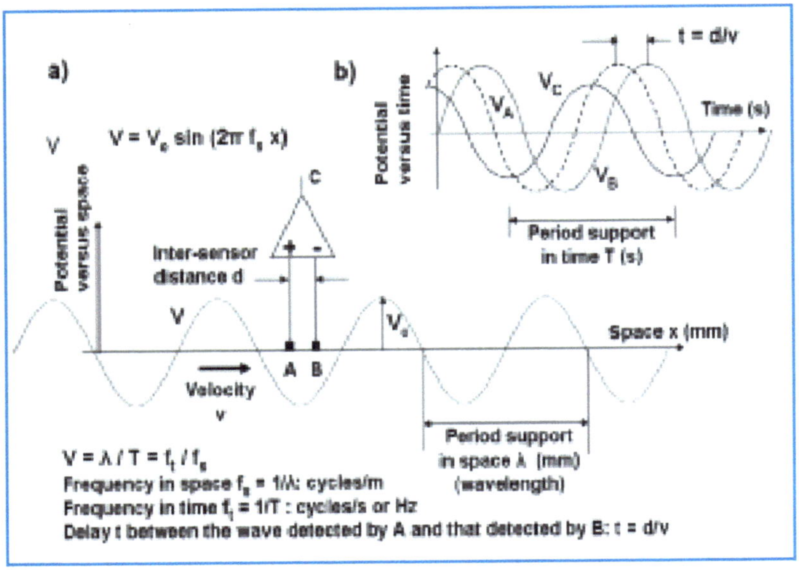


**Fig. 2.6** **a** A periodic wave in space, with amplitude Vo, wavelength λ, and spatial frequency 1/λ, is propagated, like a sea wave under two detectors, A and B. The wave $V_A$ (in time) is detected by sensor A and the waveform $V_B$ by sensor B with a delay t = d/v with respect to $V_A$. **b** Their difference, $V_C = V_A - V_B$, is computed. The relation between variables in space and time is evident

when $V_A = V_B$, as observed in previous examples.

Several important observations can be made based on Fig. 2.6. The support of a cycle in space is λ meters (wavelength) and a period in time is T seconds: this means that it takes T seconds for V to move λ meters, and the velocity is therefore v = λ/T. Therefore it takes t = d/v seconds to cover the distance of d meters, that is, the spacing between sensors A and B. $V_A$ and $V_B$ are sine waves with the same amplitude $V_o$ and the same frequency 1/T Hz (where T = λ/v) but are "out of phase" (that is, $V_B$ is delayed by t = d/v seconds with respect to $V_A$). Their difference is $V_C$, which is also a sine wave with the same frequency of $V_A$ and $V_B$ (sums or differences of sine waves of the same frequency are sine waves with the same frequency). The amplitude of $V_C$ depends on d and λ. Since, in this case, d is fixed, the amplitude of $V_C$ will depend on the wavelength λ, that is, on the spatial frequency $f_s = 1/\lambda$ of V. A device that differentially treats its input sine waves depending on their frequencies is called a "filter." If V has a spatial frequency $f_s = 1/d$, then $V_C$ is zero; if V has a spatial frequency $f_s = 1/(2d)$, that is, λ = 2d, then $V_C$ is a sine wave with an amplitude equal to $2V_o$. If $d << \lambda$, then $V_C$ is small and proportional to the derivative of V with respect to space. The reader is invited to verify these as well as other conditions and other combinations of values of d with respect to λ, and therefore to see how different input frequencies of V are treated differently by the "filter" (depicted as a triangle in Fig. 2.6a) that computes $V_C = V_A - V_B$. These concepts are very important for understanding the features of sEMG that will be described in Sects. 5.3 and 5.4.

## 2.6 A Moving Dipole Source and Two Sensors

Figure 2.7a depicts two identical sources of opposite sign, 1 and 2, at the same distance h from the surface and at a distance S from each other (for example two lights of different colors or two charges, one positive and one negative). Source 1 generates a potential profile indicated as 1 and source 2 a profile indicated as 2 and of opposite sign. The sum of the two profiles in space is indicated as 3. A pair of nearby opposite sources is indicated as a dipole.

The two sources forming the dipole move at the same velocity v to the right and their joint potential in space moves at the same velocity, passing under detector A and then under detector B but separated by a distance d. This generates the potential profiles in time $V_A$ and $V_B$ and their difference $V_C$, as explained in the previous sections and figures and depicted in Fig. 2.7b.

A dipole is often indicated schematically with two opposite arrows whose lengths represent the intensity of the sources and whose distance is equal to that separating the sources, as indicated in Fig. 2.7a.

The reader should now be able to draw the potential profiles $V_A$ and $V_B$ and their difference $V_C$ for various cases: when $d << S$, when $d = S$, when $d >> S$, and when the locations of the sources are reversed, reaching conclusions regarding how such profiles reflect the geometric parameters of the system.

## 2.7 Other Moving Sources and Multiple Sensors Aligned with the Movement Direction

Let us now consider a more complex situation, one that closely represents a schematic and simplified representation of an AP propagating along a muscle fiber. The generation and propagation of an AP are described in Chapter 3; the examples provided in Figs. 2.8 – 2.10 greatly help in understanding these concepts.

Consider the dipole depicted in Fig. 2.7. Its potential distribution is described in Fig. 2.8a as the surface halo of two lights of equal intensity (one red and one blue) at a distance S from each other and at the same depth h below the surface of a medium (such as water). Their potential distribution along the x axis is depicted in Fig. 2.8b, where the sources are also represented by two arrows, as is usual practice for a dipole. Consider now two additional smaller sources (3 and 4) forming another dipole, with source 3 coinciding with (and adding to) source 2. For clarity, in Fig. 2.8c source 3 is shown in darker blue than source 2. The strength (arrow length) of source 3 is added to that of source 2 so that the double dipole be-

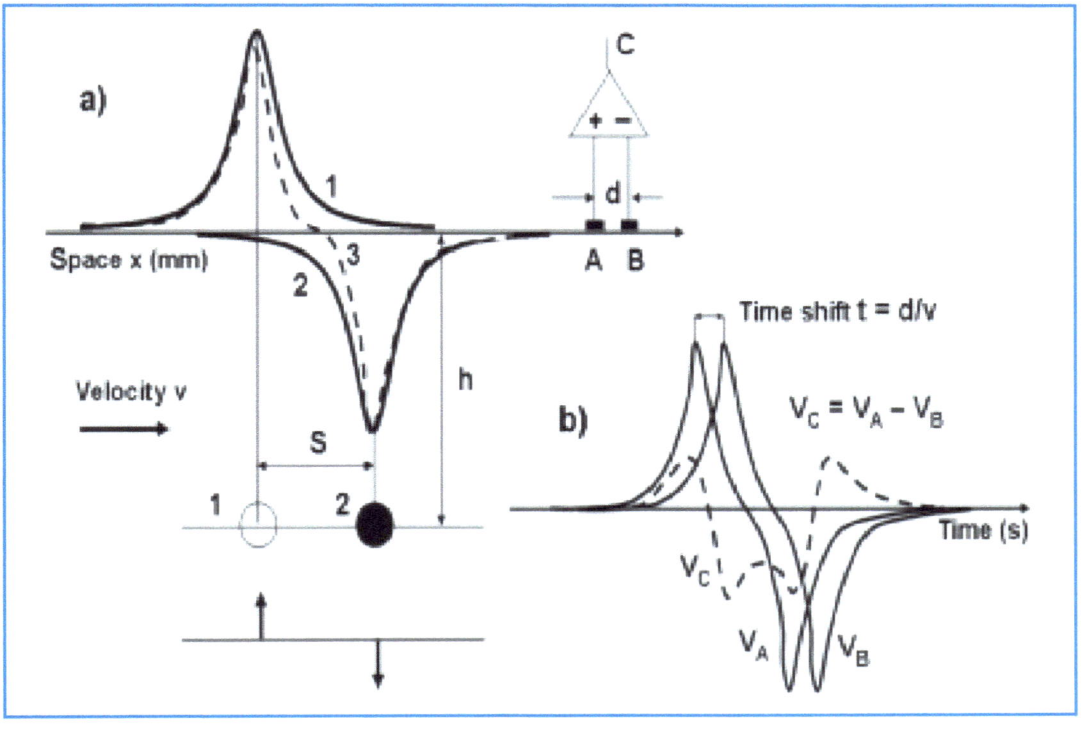


**Fig. 2.7** **a** Two sources of opposite sign (e.g., one positive and one negative, or one blue and one red, etc.), denoted as 1 and 2, are separated by a distance S and at the same depth h below a surface. Their respective potential profiles are also denoted as 1 and 2, and their sum as 3. The waveform 3 propagates, in space along the x axis, with velocity v, and passes under the two detectors A and B, generating the profiles $V_A$ and $V_B$, delayed by $t = d/v$, whose difference is $V_C$. **b** The potential profiles $V_A$, $V_B$, and $V_C = V_A - V_B$ are displayed vs. time. See also Fig. 2.8

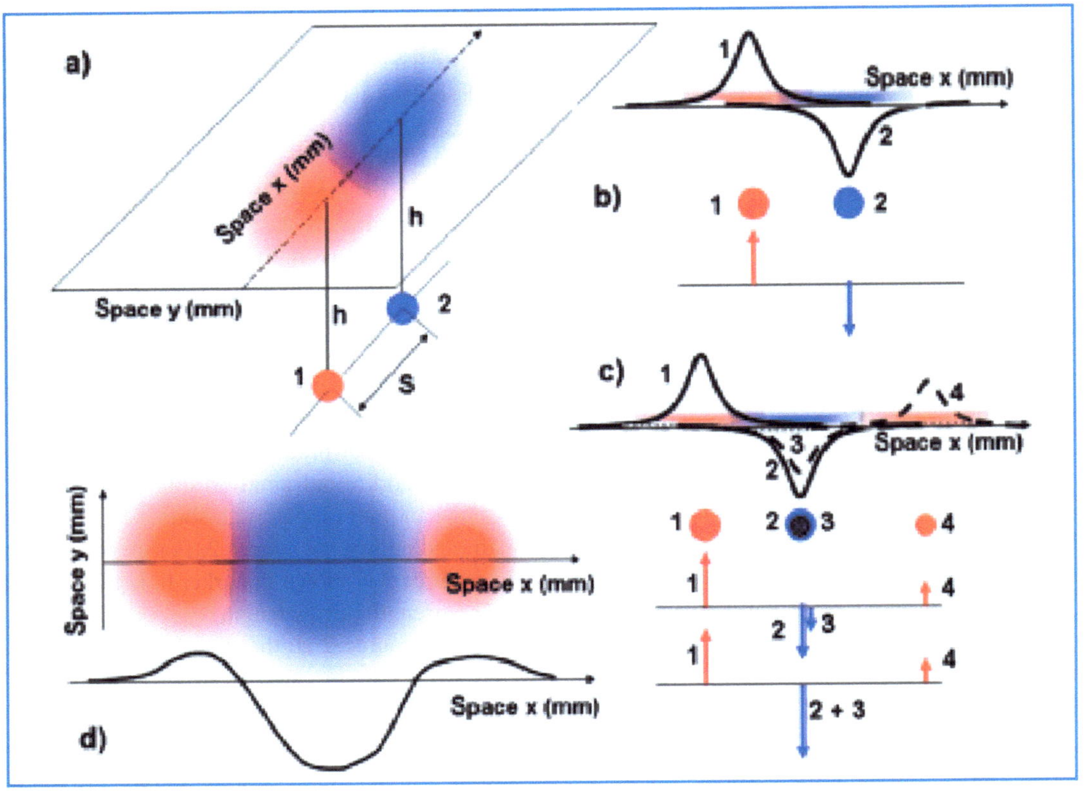


**Fig. 2.8** **a** The two sources (1 and 2) represented in Fig. 2.7a are depicted with their surface halo (potential distribution) in three dimensions. **b** The two potential profiles along the x axis are shown together with their dipole representation. **c** A second dipole is added (sources 3 and 4) with source 3 overlapping source 2. The corresponding four potential profiles (1–4) are shown with the two dipoles that, since sources 2 and 3 overlap, form a tripole. **d** The potential distribution on the x-y plane and the potential intensity along the x axis

comes a tripole (three sources whose sum is zero). The potential profiles in space of the four sources are labeled 1, 2, 3, and 4 in Fig. 2.8c. The surface halo of this tripole (as an example, with red and blue lights) is depicted in Fig. 2.8d together with the potential profile along the x axis. The reader is invited to investigate the waveforms $V_A$, $V_B$, and $V_C$ resulting in time if the tripole of Fig. 2.8 moves under the detection system depicted in Fig. 2.7. As illustrated in Chapter 3, a moving tripole is a good approximation of an AP propagating along a muscle fiber.

Consider now the tripole depicted in Fig. 2.8c and its potential profile in space along the x axis on the surface above it (Fig. 2.8d). Consider also the monopolar detection system depicted in Fig. 2.4 and suppose that we have 16 equally spaced detectors (A–P in Fig. 2.9a) and providing 16 outputs (1–16) measured with respect to a remote reference at zero potential. At a specific time instant $t_o$, the sensors provide 16 samples of the potential profile in space. These samples are taken d mm apart from each other, where d is the inter-sensor distance. They are indicated with thick vertical lines under the potential profile, below the 16 sensors. The outputs of the system are $V_1 = V_A$, $V_2 = V_B$, .....,$V_{16} = V_P$.

If the sources generating the potential profile are moving with velocity v along a line parallel to the surface and to the sensor array, each sensor will detect a potential profile in time, as indicated in Fig. 2.4. Each of these potentials in time will reproduce the shape of the potential in space and will be delayed by $t = d/v$ with respect to the previous

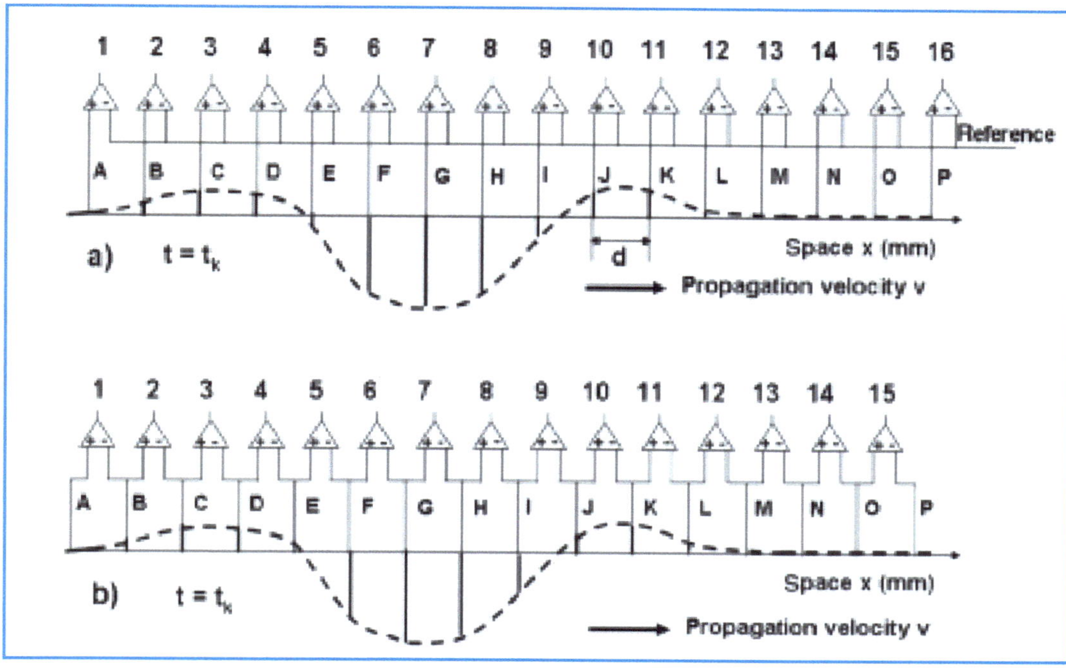


**Fig. 2.9** **a** Array of 16 aligned and equally spaced detectors (A–P) providing 16 monopolar outputs, i.e., 16 instantaneous and simultaneous samples of the underlying potential profile. **b** Array of 16 aligned and equally spaced detectors (A–P) providing 15 differential outputs; that is, 15 instantaneous and simultaneous samples of the differences VA – VB, VB – VC....VO – VP. If the potential profile moves, each of the outputs 1–16 or 1–15 is a function of time (see Fig. 2.10)

one. The result will be the generation of the 16 time waveforms depicted in Fig. 2.10. Figure 2.9b shows the configuration for the differential detection of the potential distribution along x. The basic concept was explained in Figs. 2.5 and 2.6. In this case, the outputs of the system will be: $V_1 = V_A - V_B$, $V_2 = V_B - V_C$ .....,$V_{15} = V_O - V_P$.

Additional issues and questions can now be addressed: for example, can the reader draw the differential profiles, obtained from Fig. 2.9b, in time? If the vertical grid lines in Fig. 2.10 are 5 ms apart and the sensors are 10 mm apart, what is the velocity of the sources? What would the monopolar and the differential potentials profiles in time look like if the conduction velocity was in the opposite direction? How would the monopolar and differential potentials be modified if the + and – signs of each detector system were reversed? What is the profile position in Fig. 2.9a that corresponds to the first, second, etc., time division of Fig. 2.10?As an additional exercise, label the time divisions of Fig. 2.10 for d = 10 mm and v = 4 m/s.

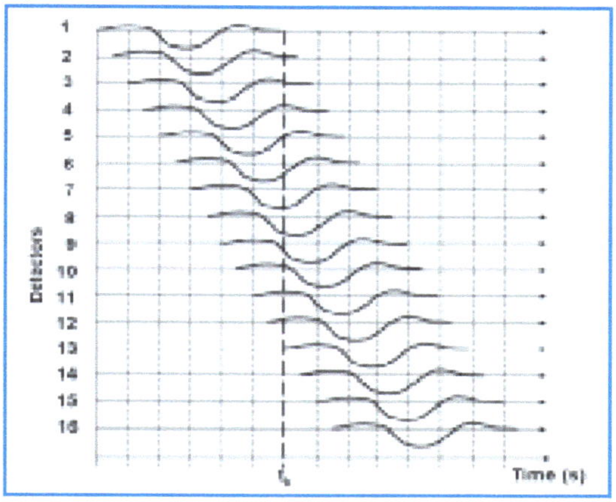


**Fig. 2.10** Example of the 16 outputs of the detection system of Fig. 2.9a when the potential profile moves in space, from top to bottom, at constant velocity v. The potential first appears under detector A (output 1), then B, etc. and finally under P (output 16). Each time trace is delayed from the preceding one by a time given by d/v. The time instant $t_k$ depicted in Fig. 2.9a is outlined. The samples of the array of potentials at time $t_k$ are the same as those depicted in Fig. 2.9a and they provide the representation of the potential distribution in space at this particular time instant

## 2.8 Grids of Detectors and Two-Dimensional Representations

Let us now apply, on the surface of the medium, a series of detector arrays parallel to each other and equally spaced so that a rectangular grid of detectors is obtained, as represented by the circles in Fig. 2.11a. The circles are equally spaced in both directions, x and y and identify small squares that are referred to as picture elements, or pixels. The grid (or matrix) depicted in Fig. 2.11a has 65 pixels. The detector has an area over which the potential is averaged. This mean value is the potential value of the pixel so that the pixels appear as squares of uniform intensity. Consider now a two-dimensional (2D) potential distribution such as that generated by a tripole and depicted in Fig. 2.8d as a distribution of red and blue lights (or positive and negative potentials) in space. As shown in Chapter 3, this distribution is a reasonable representation of a muscle fiber AP.

Applying the grid of detectors to this type of potential distribution (as shown in Fig. 2.11a) yields the image shown in Fig. 2.11b. It is obvious that the finer the grid the more accurate the representation of the potential distribution. However, if the representation provided in Fig. 2.11b is detected with a "fine enough" grid, then the much finer original picture can be reconstructed by a mathematical process called "interpolation." The definition of a "fine enough" grid is related to the concept underlying the sampling theorem in space, a discussion of which is beyond the scope of this book.

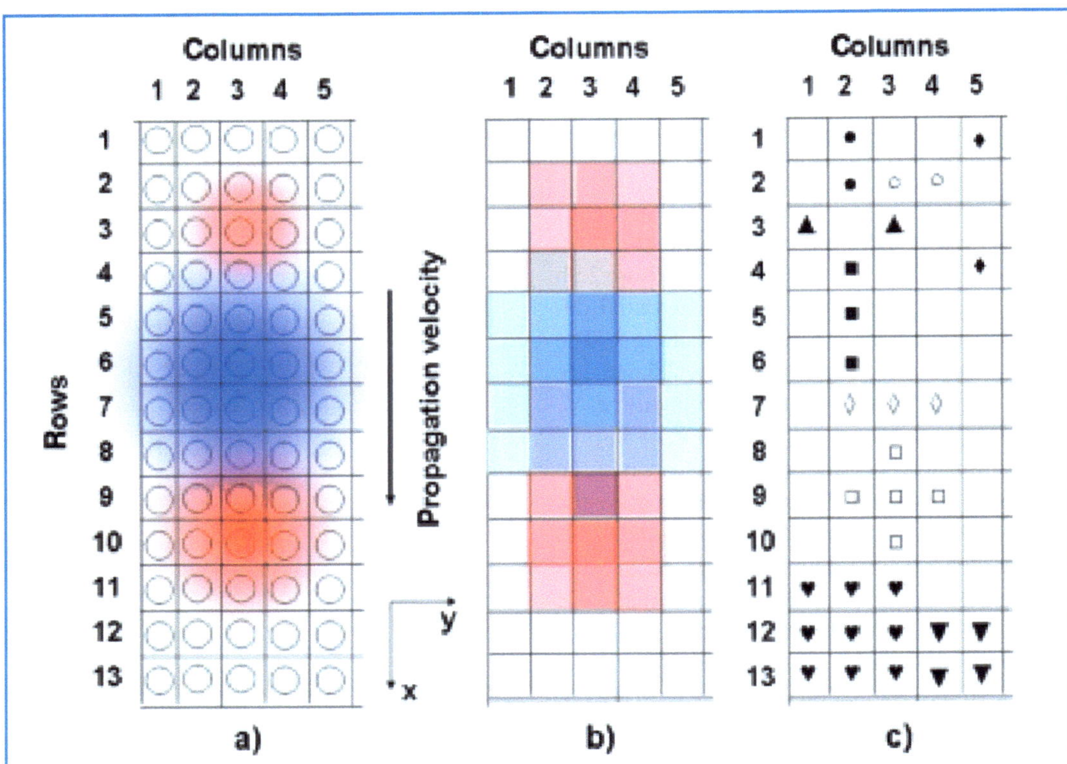


**Fig. 2.11** **a** A 13 × 5 two-dimensional (2D) grid of detectors superimposed on a 2D potential distribution. **b** A representation of the potential distribution as 13 × 5 pixels. **c** Examples of spatial filters: ● Longitudinal single differential with one interdetector distance: ◆ longitudinal single differential with three interdetector distances; ○ transversal single differential with one interdetector distance; ▲ transversal single differential with two interdetector distances; ■ longitudinal double differential; ◊ transversal double differential; □ Laplacian filter (see text) ♥ and ▼ other filters (see text)

Let us now assume that the potential distribution is moving under the grid with constant velocity v. This condition was already investigated in the case of a single array (Figs. 2.9, 2.10). The detectors aligned with the direction of movement form the columns and those aligned in the perpendicular direction form the rows, as indicated in Fig. 2.11a, b. Each linear array (column) will detect signals similar to those depicted in Fig. 2.10. Columns that are lateral with respect to the sources will detect smaller signals. The reader is invited to imagine the signals appearing on the grid for a tripole source either very close to the surface or deep (consider Fig. 2.3 as a guideline). Also, imagine a tripole source propagating along a direction not aligned with the columns of the grid.

A full understanding of potential maps evolving in space and time for different sources (monopole, dipole, tripole) propagating in directions not necessarily aligned with the columns of the grid is of great importance for the interpretation of sEMG images and movies. Movies of the potentials evolving in time and space can be downloaded from the website http://extras.springer.com.

## 2.9 The Concept of a Spatial Filter

Certain samples (pixel intensities) of the potential distribution in space may be combined by adding them after multiplication of each one by a given "weight." This process of "linear combination" was already shown in Figure 2.5 for the simple case of two detection points "weighted" with weights equal to 1 and – 1, so that their difference is obtained by the summation of these weighted versions. The output of a spatial filter can be interpreted either as a pixel of a new "filtered" image or as a signal varying in time and resulting from the filtering operation performed in space.

Figure 2.5d showed how a totally different waveform ($V_C$) is obtained by adding the outputs of two detectors, $V_A$ and $-V_B$. Consider now the grid of detectors shown in Fig. 2.11c and let us label the single pixels with the row subscript followed by the column subscript so that the pixel in the upper left corner has a potential $V_{1,1}$, that in the upper right corner $V_{1,5}$, that in the lower left corner $V_{13,1}$ and that in the lower right corner $V_{13,5}$. Consider the difference, in the column direction $V_{1,2} - V_{2,2}$ (black circles). This is similar to $V_C = V_A - V_B$ in Fig. 2.5d and is referred to as a longitudinal differential recording. This recording modality may be extended along the column, as in Fig. 2.9b, so that a sequence of longitudinal differential recordings is obtained. Consider now the difference $V_{1,5} - V_{4,5}$ (black diamonds). This is also a longitudinal differential recording but the distance between the chosen detectors is three inter-detector distances instead of one.

The same can be done in the transversal direction. For example, $V_{2,3} - V_{2,4}$ (empty circles) is a transversal differential recording with one inter-detector distance, while $V_{3,1} - V_{3,3}$ (black up triangles) is also a transversal differential recording with two inter-detector distances.

Consider now the double difference $(V_{4,2} - V_{5,2}) - (V_{5,} - V_{6,2}) = V_{4,2} - 2V_{5,2} + V_{6,2}$ (black squares) where $V_{4,2}$ is assigned weight 1, $V_{5,2}$ is assigned weight – 2 and $V_{6,2}$ is assigned weight 1. This is called a "longitudinal double differential recording."

The double difference $(V_{7,2} - V_{7,3})$ - $(V_{7,3} - V_{7,4}) = V_{7,2} - 2V_{7,3} + V_{7,4}$ (white diamonds) is called a "transversal double differential recording." The combination of a longitudinal and a transversal double differential detection forms a Laplacian filter, defined in the example of Fig. 2.11c by $V_{8,3} + V_{9,2} + V_{9,4} + V_{10,3} - 4\,V_{9,3}$ having weights – 4 for the central detector and 1 for the other four detectors.

Other filters may be designed: for example, the 3 × 3 filter depicted with black hearts could have the weight – 8 for $V_{12,2}$ and 1 for the other eight potentials or weight – 12 for $V_{12,2}$ , 2 for the pixels above and below, right and left, and 1 for the four pixels in diagonal positions. It should be observed that the sum of the weights is always zero. This is important in "differential" filters in order to eliminate the contribution of "common mode potentials," which are identical under all detectors. The filters involving at least three detectors enhance the potential under one detector (the central one) and subtract the potentials of the surrounding electrodes, thereby enhancing sharp spatial peaks, attenuating slow spatial changes, and removing components common to all detectors. "Single differential" or "bipolar" detection systems also remove any common component but do not have a detector as a center of symmetry: their center of symmetry is between two detectors.

Another type of filters averages the potentials under adjacent detectors and creates an equivalent larger detector that, in the example of Fig. 2.11c (black inverted triangles), collects the potential $(V_{12,4} + V_{12,5} + V_{13,4} + V_{13,5})/4$. In this case, any common component remains unchanged.

Differential spatial filters are used to "focus" the detection in a specific region of space and to attenuate contributions from lateral and deeper sources: they act as "focusing devices" limiting the "detection volume" of the system. Of course, they can be applied to a group of pixels and then, iteratively, along successive columns of detectors until the entire grid is covered. This produces a longitudinal single differential map, a longitudinal double differential map, a longitudinal Laplacian map, etc. The applications, advantages, and disadvantages of these spatial filtering operations in the case of sEMG are described in Chapter 4 and, more extensively, in the literature (Reucher et al. 1987a, 1987b).

## Suggested Reading

Reucher H, Rau G, Silny J (1987a) Spatial filtering of noninvasive multielectrode EMG: Part I - Introduction to measuring technique and applications. IEEE Trans Biomed Eng 34:98-105

Reucher H, Silny J, Rau G (1987b) Spatial filtering of noninvasive multielectrode EMG: Part II - Filter performance in theory and modeling. IEEE Trans Biomed Eng 34:106-13

# Generation, Propagation, and Extinction of Single-Fiber and Motor Unit Action Potentials

3


**Abstract**

This chapter addresses the issue of associating the location and nature of the electric field sources below the surface of a conductive medium with the corresponding potential distribution on that surface. Single-point sources (monopoles), pairs of opposite sources (dipoles), and pairs of dipoles (tripoles or quadrupoles) are investigated together with the detection modalities of the surface potential (monopolar, differential, etc.). The electric potentials generated by sources moving under these detection systems are described using a qualitative approach. The general concept of a spatial filter is introduced.


## 3.1 The Membrane Resting Potential

Consider a small patch of membrane of a muscle fiber, as indicated in Fig. 3.1a. The membrane resembles a sieve, permeable to water and, in varying degrees, also to sodium ($Na^+$), potassium ($K^+$), chlorine ($Cl^-$), and other, less relevant positive and negative ions present outside and inside the muscle fiber. The permeability to each ion is due to pore-like channels in the membrane. These channels have very interesting properties. Firstly, they are selective, that is, there are sodium channels, potassium channels, etc., and they can open or close depending on the difference in electric potential across the membrane (membrane voltage). Secondly, a fundamental feature of the membrane is a pumping mechanism (active transport), pumping $Na^+$ ions out and $K^+$ ions in. These pumps are indicated with thick arrows in Fig. 3.1b.

The operation of these pumps increases the concentration of $Na^+$ ions outside and $K^+$ ions inside the muscle fiber. Of course, $Na^+$ and $K^+$ ions partially flow back through the respective channels because of the concentration gradients created by the pumps. These flows are indicated with thin arrows in Fig. 3.1b. Ions are electrically charged and their concentration difference generates an electric potential difference with the positive pole, where there is a surplus of positive charges, and with the negative pole, where there is a surplus of negative charges. The two pumps do not balance each other. For this and other reasons (not discussed in this book) the inside of the cell is negative with respect to the outside, creating a potential gradient (electric field) across the membrane. The concept of potential was introduced in Chapter 1. Both $Na^+$ ions and $K^+$ ions are positive and therefore move from the positive region outside the cell to the negative region inside the cell. Their flows due to the potential gradient are indicated with dashed arrows in Fig. 3.1b. By contrast, chlorine ions are negative and flow from the negative region inside the cell to the positive region outside the cell. This creates an accumulation of $Cl^-$ ions outside and therefore a flow along the concentration gradient, returning a fraction of the $Cl^-$ ions.

These flows eventually reach a balance point when, over a unit time, equal numbers of $Na^+$ ions enter and exit the membrane as do equal numbers of $K^+$ ions. The same holds true for $Cl^-$ ions. This equilib-


M. Barbero, R. Merletti, A. Rainoldi, *Atlas of Muscle Innervation Zones*,

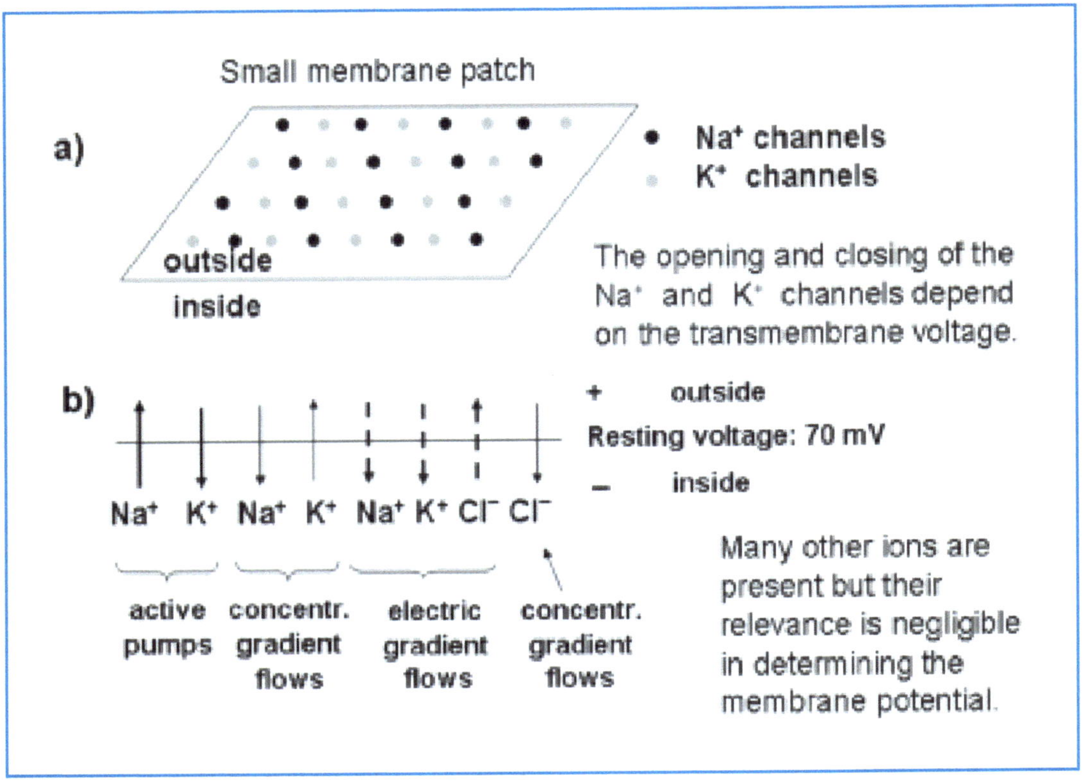


**Fig. 3.1** **a** A patch of muscle cell membrane showing $Na^+$ and $K^+$ channels. $Cl^-$ channels are also present but are not indicated. All channels are voltage dependent and may open to a greater or lesser extent depending on the membrane voltage. **b** The horizontal line indicates a patch of membrane. *Arrows* indicate ion flows: *thick arrows* indicate the active transport of $Na^+$ and $K^+$ ions, *thin arrows* flows along a concentration gradient, *dashed arrows* flows along the electric potential gradient (the electric field). Equilibrium is reached when the outgoing flow equals the ingoing flow for each ion. This condition implies the generation of a 70 mV resting membrane potential, with the negative pole inside and the positive pole outside

rium condition is reached when the voltage across the membrane is 70 mV, with the negative pole inside the cell and the positive pole outside. Note that the "net" flow is zero for each ion in this condition but each of the three flows of $Na^+$ and $K^+$ ions and each of the two flows of $Cl^-$ ions is not zero. When this equilibrium condition is reached, the voltage across the membrane is indicated as the resting membrane voltage, or the resting membrane potential. There is only one equilibrium condition, corresponding to a voltage of 70 mV, with the negative pole inside and the positive pole outside. Maintaining this condition requires energy because the pumps are pumping ions against their concentration gradients, like pumping water up a hill against gravity. Dead cells do not have any resting potential.

## 3.2 Generation of the Action Potential

Let us now consider the short section of a tubular cell, as depicted in Fig. 3.2a and indicated as $\alpha$, and its resting membrane potential of – 70 mV. Suppose that an external "stimulus" (e.g., a chemical, such as a neurotransmitter) locally increases membrane permeability to $Na^+$ ions (by opening up a few of the $Na^+$ channels). Of course, $Na^+$ ions will rush into the cell, following their concentration gradient. If this disturbance is sufficiently small and momentary, the cell membrane recovers and its voltage returns to the resting value (phase 1 in Fig. 3.2b, c). If this disturbance is stronger or longer, the inflow

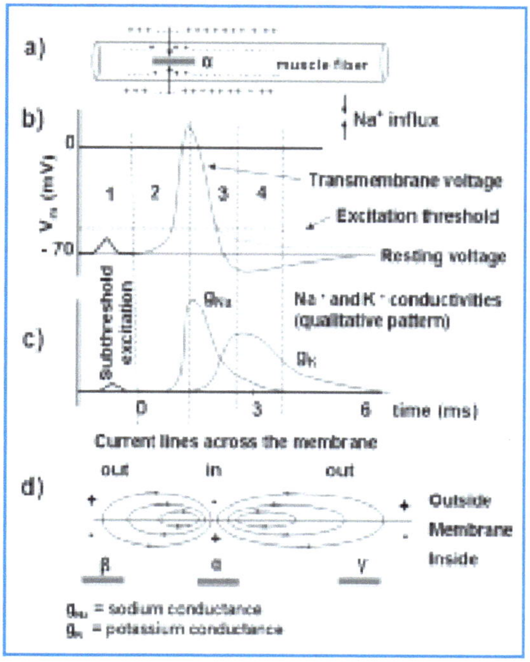


**Fig. 3.2** A cylindrical muscle cell (**a**) with resting potential of –70 mV. Region α is disturbed by a small increase in $Na^+$ conductivity ($g_{Na}$ and $g_K$ = ionic conductivities = electrical equivalents to membrane permeabilities to $Na^+$ and $K^+$ ions) insufficient to trigger an action potential (AP) (phase 1) or by a larger increase in which the excitation threshold is crossed, generating the depolarization phase (phase 2) of an AP. **b, c** Representation of the membrane voltage (AP) of region α vs. time (**b**) and of the membrane conductivities (permeabilities) to $Na^+$ and $K^+$ ions during the AP (**c**). **d** Current flows near region α caused by the AP and resulting in the depolarization of nearby regions β and γ (see Sect. 3.3 for details)

of $Na^+$ will be sufficient to modify the membrane voltage to an extent that an "excitation threshold" is crossed (Fig. 3.2b), beyond which the voltage change induces a greater increase in $Na^+$ permeability so that $Na^+$ ions increasingly rush in and further raise the membrane voltage towards zero. This, in turn, increases the permeability to $Na^+$ ions even further, such that the flow to the inside additionally raises the membrane voltage. This positive feedback is self-sustaining and evolves rapidly until the $Na^+$ channels are completely open (phase 2 in Fig. 3.2b, c). At this point, the membrane voltage is about + 20–30 mV (positive inside and negative outside). In the meantime, but with some delay, a shift of the membrane voltage toward zero causes the opening of the $K^+$ channels (which are also voltage dependent), increasing the permeability to $K^+$ ions, which rush out following their concentration gradient. The outflow of positive charges counteracts the potential increase due to the inflow of $Na^+$ ions, so that the membrane voltage starts to fall toward zero. Consequently, there is less permeability to $Na^+$ ions, the $Na^+$ channels begin to close, and the membrane voltage drops further, reversing the events of phase 2. This self-sustaining process continues until the membrane voltage returns to the resting value, at which point the permeabilities to both $Na^+$ and $K^+$ ions return to the respective resting values (phase 3 in Fig. 3.2b). The return may take place with an undershoot (as indicated in phase 4, Fig. 3.2b, solid line), due to the slower dynamics of the permeability to $K^+$ ions, or with a tail lasting a few tens of milliseconds, depending on the interplay of the $K^+$ and $Na^+$ permeabilities (as indicated in phase 4, Fig. 3.2b, dotted line). When this transient is terminated, the original membrane condition is restored and the membrane voltage is again at its resting value of – 70 mV.

The entire process, once started, evolves as described without the need of additional inputs, nor is it responsive to additional external events (refractory period).

An electrical analogy of this phenomenon is a "one shot" circuit. A mechanical-hydraulic analogy is the triggered flushing and automatic refilling of the water tank of a toilet.

The entire time event (phases 2, 3, and 4) is called an "action potential" (AP) and in a muscle cell it lasts about 4–6 ms (excluding a possible slow long tail). The above description of an AP refers to the evolution *in time* of both the ionic permeabilities and the membrane voltage in a small patch of membrane of a cylindrical cell. What happens during this time in the nearby membrane patches is described in the following section.

## 3.3 Propagation of the Action Potential

Let us now consider what happens in the nearby patches of membrane when the voltage in patch α is at its peak (end of phase 2 and beginning of phase 3, in Fig. 3.2b, c). Figure. 3.2d shows the distribution of electric current *in space* along the outside and inside of the membrane at the time of the AP peak. Moving from left to right, we see a region β, where the membrane voltage has its normal polarity; a region α, where the polarity is momentarily reversed; and a region γ, where the polarity is again normal. Since the intracellular and extracellular fluids are electrically conductive, currents flow from positive regions to negative regions, that is from α to β outside the cell and from β to α inside the cell, creating loops as indicated between the α and β regions in Fig. 3.2d. The same happens between regions α and γ. The information is similarly provided in Fig. 3.3, where batteries represent the local membrane voltage at time instant $t_0$.

We can then observe that currents cross the membrane from inside to outside in regions β and γ. These currents modify the membrane voltage such that it is less negative. The voltage change is sufficient to increase the membrane voltage above the excitation threshold so that an AP is generated in both regions. The patch α, where the membrane voltage is momentarily reversed (peak of the AP waveform in Fig. 3.2b), therefore widens in space and involves a progressively longer segment of the fiber, extending to patches β and γ. Of course,

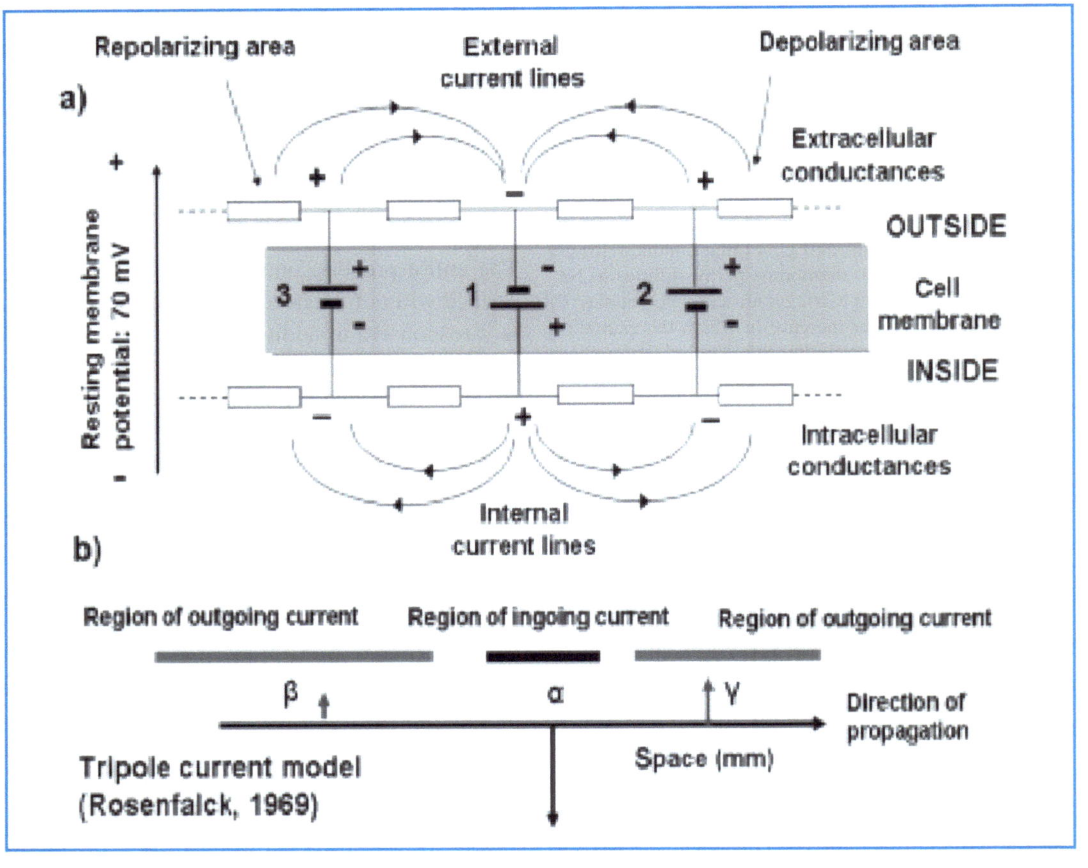


**Fig. 3.3** **a** Representation of the AP in space at a given time $t_0$ (see Fig. 3.2a, d). Battery 1 represents the region of peak membrane depolarization, battery 2 the region in which the depolarization is taking place (corresponding to time interval 2 in Fig. 3.2), and battery 3 the region of repolarization (corresponding to time interval 3 in Fig. 3.2). Note the dualism between the two representations of the AP in time and space (see also Fig. 2.4). These voltages in space create a distribution of current across the membrane that moves, like a wave, in a longitudinal direction, along the cell (see Figs. 2.4–2.7). **b** Tripole representation of the ingoing current (*downward arrow*) and outgoing currents (*upward arrows*). The tripole moves to the right and the voltage across each point of the membrane evolves in time, as indicated in Fig. 3.2b

this phenomenon also extends to the left of β and to the right of γ, causing a further widening region of the membrane "depolarization." As this happens, patch α "repolarizes," as described in phases 3 and 4 of Fig. 3.2b, and returns to the normal membrane condition. It should now be clear that the sequence of events in time and space described in Fig. 3.2 can be summarized as follows and as described in Figs. 3.3 and 3.4:

1. In a small patch α of the membrane, a local AP is triggered either by an external chemical (Fig. 3.2) or by the electrical action of a contiguous patch (Fig. 3.3). The membrane depolarizes, that is, the polarity of its potential is momentarily reversed.
2. The depolarization rapidly widens in space (patches β and γ and beyond) while patch α repolarizes to the original resting condition (Fig. 3.2d).
3. The original region of depolarization splits into two regions that move, respectively, to the right and left of the point of origin with a certain velocity, like the waves that are formed when a stone has been dropped into a long and narrow pool of water.

Figure 3.3a schematically shows an AP (generated outside the figure) moving from left to right. The local membrane potentials are represented by batteries. Battery 1 represents the repolarizing region (tail of the AP), battery 2 the depolarized region (peak of the AP), and battery 3 the depolarizing region (front of the AP). The arrows represent the currents that flow in and out of the cell through the membrane. These currents may be assumed, for simplicity, to enter or exit the cell at one point each rather than in a region: with this approximation, they can be represented as three arrows whose sum is zero, as indicated in Figs. 3.3b and 3.4.

Figure 3.4a, c, and e depict the events that take place in time and space around the circumference of the cell. They show cylindrical symmetry. As indicated in Fig. 3.3b, these events can be modeled as being due to point sources of current.

The current entering the cell can be represented as a downwards arrow, with its length representing the current intensity and its position the point of entry (which is the centroid of the region of entry). Similarly, the current exiting the cell can be represented as an upwards arrow. Since a propagating AP shows a region of ingoing current and two regions of outgoing current, the AP can be represented in space by a current tripole. Figure 3.4f shows the two current tripoles that schematically represent the two APs propagating in opposite directions, as depicted in Fig. 3.4e. The mechanism resulting in the progressive generation of these two current tripoles is shown in Fig. 3.4a–d. These currents flow in the extracellular space and produce potential distributions on the surface of the skin, as indicated in Fig. 2.8c, d.

Another way of describing AP generation and propagation phenomena is to consider the positively and negatively charged extracellular regions

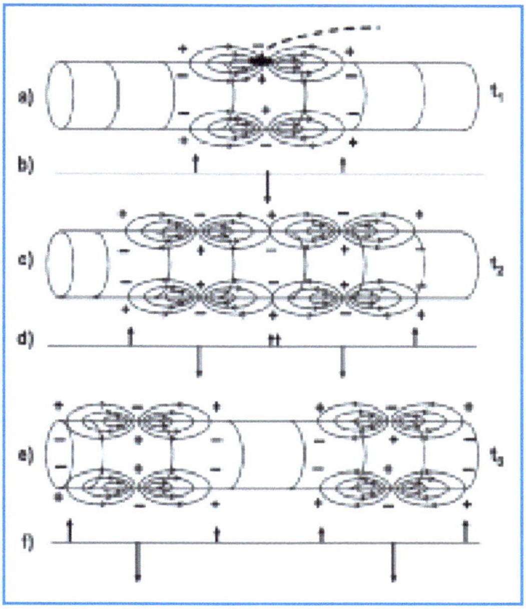


**Fig. 3.4** Generation and propagation of an AP in a cylindrical muscle fiber. **a** The dashed line is an axonal branch releasing acetylcholine at the neuromuscular junction, thereby increasing the local permeability to $Na^+$ ions and triggering the AP. The underlying membrane depolarizes, as described in Fig. 3.2, generating current loops that depolarize nearby regions of the cells. **b** The current "poles" corresponding to this situation at time $t_1$ are depicted. **c** Two APs are being generated in space as the original area repolarizes. **d** The current "poles" corresponding to this situation at time $t_2$ are depicted: two tripoles are generated. **e** The two APs are fully generated and travel in opposite directions. **f** Two separate current tripoles describe the propagating APs at time $t_3$. Conditions **a**, **c**, and **e** are captured at time instants $t_1$, $t_2$, and $t_3$

(indicated as + – + in Figs. 3.2–3.4) generated (and propagating) in space by each AP as a tripole of electrical charges producing an electric field in the surrounding conductive volume and a potential distribution on the skin surface, just as described in Fig. 2.8.

It can be shown that in either case the tripole source actually comprises two dipoles with two overlapping sources, as previously described in Fig. 2.8c, d. The sum of the currents that generate the potential is zero at any time. The two dipoles are not identical and generate fields that are in opposite directions. Consequently, their potentials partially cancel each other. The distance between the first and the third source of a tripole is about 5–10 mm and the spread of the potential distribution on the surface of the skin, in the direction of propagation, is about 10–20 mm (see Figs. 2.8 and 2.9).

Figure 3.5 shows an array of potential detectors (black dots labeled A–P) applied to the skin and amplifiers (triangles, with outputs labeled 1–16). The concepts introduced in Sect. 2.5 and Fig. 2.9, concerning the monopolar or differential detection in space of the potential generated by one or more moving sources, are now applied to interpret the monopolar and differential outputs (1–16 in Fig. 3.5a and 1–15 in Fig. 3.5e, respectively). The dashed line represents the potential distribution present on the skin surface at a given time instant $t = t_k$ and generated by the two tripoles moving to the right and left of the generation point, which is the neuromuscular junction (NMJ) or end-plate where the depolarization begins. At time $t_k$, tripole $T_1$ is under sensor D and tripole $T_2$ is under sensor M. The monopolar voltages at outputs 1–16 (Fig. 3.5a) are the samples in space, at time $t_k$, of the po-

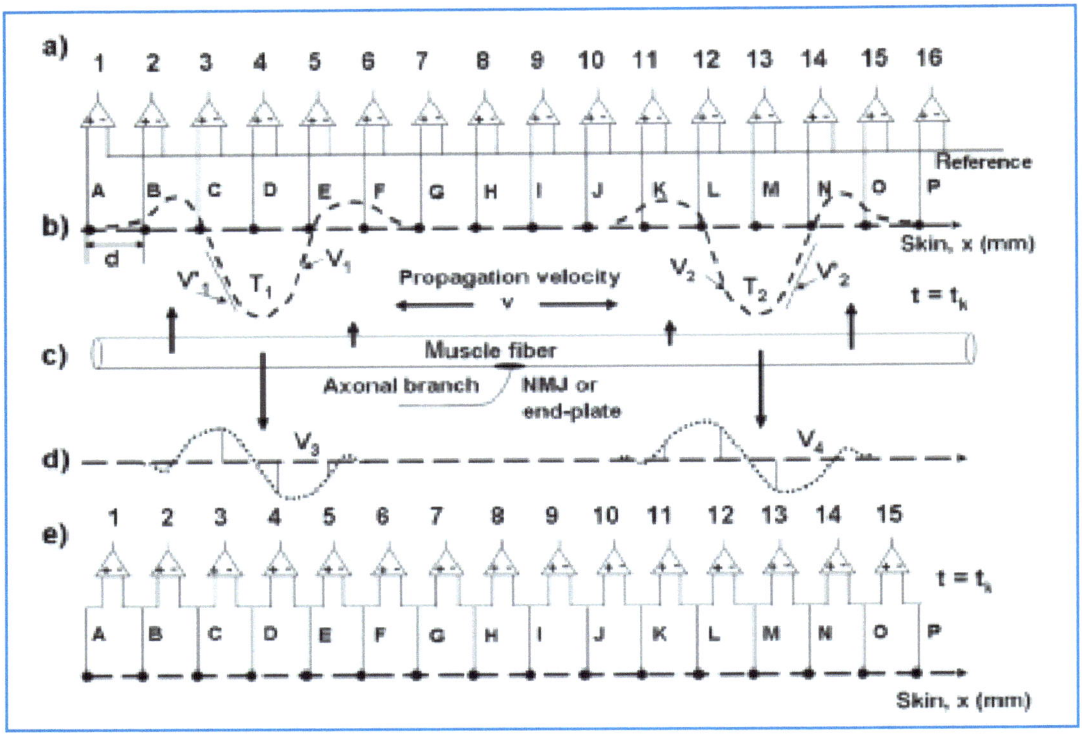


**Fig. 3.5** **a** Array of 16 monopolar amplifiers that sample the voltage (potential profile in space) with 16 detectors (electrodes placed on the skin and depicted in **b**) at any time instant $t_k$ with respect to a remote reference taken to be at zero voltage. **b** The array of electrodes and potential distributions ($V_1$ and $V_2$) generated by the two propagating tripoles ($T_1$ and $T_2$) at the time instant $t_k$ when they are, respectively, under electrode D and electrode M (see also Fig. 2.8c, d, Figs. 3.3 and 3.4; the voltage fronts $V'_1$ and $V'_2$ are discussed in Fig. 3.6) **c** A muscle fiber showing the neuromuscular junction (NMJ or end-plate) and the propagating tripoles $T_1$ and $T_2$. **d** Differential voltages taken between adjacent electrodes in the order $V_A - V_B = V_1$; $V_O - V_P = V_{15}$. **e** Electrodes and amplifiers connected in a differential configuration

tential distribution over the skin, $V_1$ and $V_2$ (Figs. 2.9a, 3.5b), measured with respect to a remote reference at zero potential.
The voltages at outputs 1–15 of Fig. 3.5e are the differences, at time $t_k$, $V_A - V_B$, $V_B - V_C$, up to $V_O - V_P$. Their continuous (analog) versions are labeled $V_3$ and $V_4$ and their samples V1–V15 in Fig. 3.5e. The voltages $V_3$ and $V_4$ and their samples are not present on the skin, they are computed by the detection system constituted by the 15 differential amplifiers, as described in Sect. 2.3 and Fig. 2.5. At any given time, the voltages present on the 16 monopolar outputs and on the 15 differential outputs of the amplifier arrays shown in Fig. 3.5a and e represent the spatial samples of $V_1$, $V_2$ and $V_3$, $V_4$. However, they evolve in time as the tripoles move and therefore generate 16 (or 15) time signals. On one side of the NMJ, the monopolar signals appear as indicated in Fig. 2.10: on the other side, they appear as a mirror reflection.
Consider now the monopolar voltages in space, $V_1$ and $V_2$ (described in Fig. 3.5b), as they move in space. $V_1$ moves to the left and $V_2$ to the right. As front $V'_1$ moves to the left it generates positive voltages on outputs 3, then 2, then 1 in Fig. 3.5e. As front $V'_2$ moves to the right, it generates negative voltages on outputs 13, then 14, then 15 in Fig. 3.5e. The same can be observed if we imagine voltages $V_3$ and $V_4$ moving, respectively, to the left and to the right.
Consequently, the differential outputs to the right of the NMJ will display, in time, first a negative and then a positive swing, whereas the differential outputs to the left of the NMJ will display, in time, first a positive and then a negative swing. The opposite occurs if the amplifiers are placed with the non-inverting input (+) to the right of the inverting input (–), so that, for example, $V_1 = V_B - V_A$ instead of $V_1 = V_A - V_B$ and so on in Fig. 3.5e. Thus, if the electrode array is reversed, all the differential signals in time will be of opposite polarity.

## 3.4 The "End-of-Fiber" Effect

The muscle fiber has a finite length and terminates at two fiber-tendon junctions. What happens to the propagating tripoles and the AP at these two ends? Different models are discussed in the literature; here we describe a simple one.
Consider the time instant $t_1$ in Fig. 3.6a, when the tripole, the corresponding current flows, and potential distributions are approaching the end of the fiber, beyond which currents cannot flow and excitation stops. Consider the two dipoles making up the tripole, dipole $D_1$ (gray arrows), and dipole $D_2$ (black arrows). Dipole $D_1$ progressively narrows (Fig. 3.6c, d) and the distance between its two poles decreases, weakening the dipole field so that its contribution to the surface potentials is reduced. When the two poles of $D_1$ overlap, they cancel out and the dipole disappears (Fig. 3.6e, f).

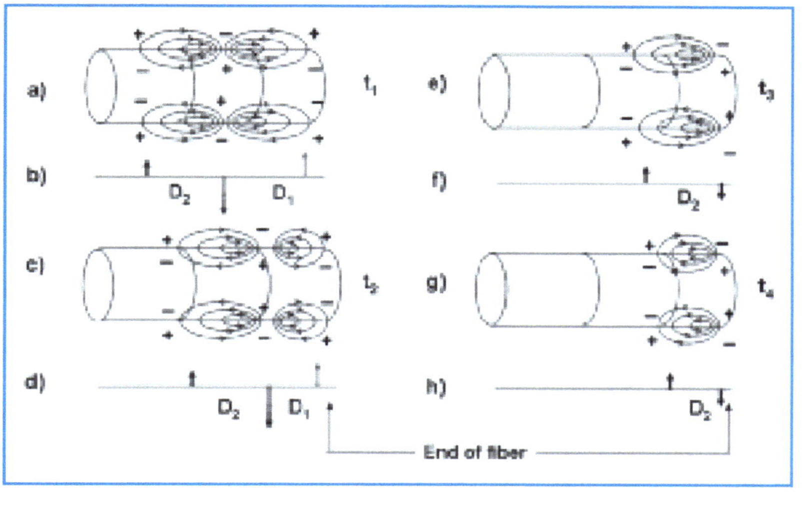


**Fig. 3.6** Extinction of the AP at the end of the fiber. **a, b** The current tripole ($D_1 + D_2$) that describes the AP approaches the fiber end. **c, d** The rightmost pole cannot go further and the dipole $D_1$ shrinks. **e, f** The two poles of dipole $D_1$ are canceled out and only dipole $D_2$ remains. **g, h** Dipole $D_2$ shrinks until the two poles cancel out and the AP is extinguished

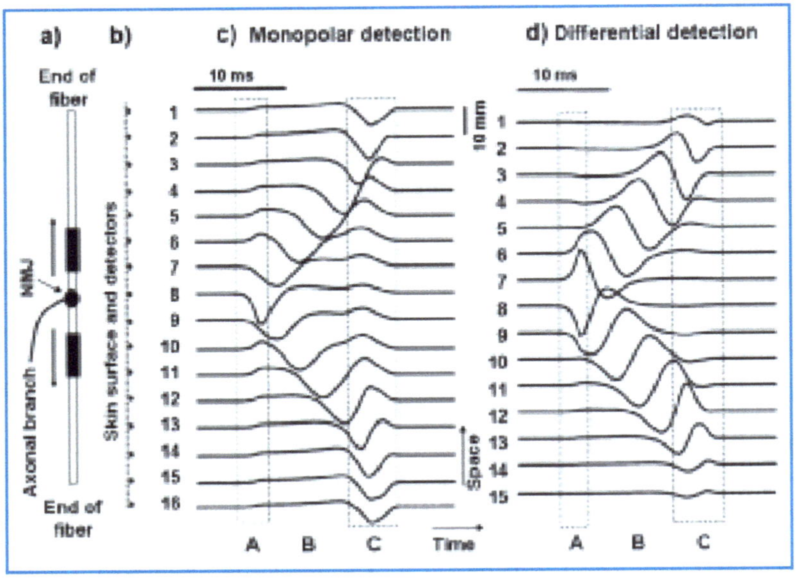


**Fig. 3.7** **a** A muscle cell of finite length, with the NMJ in the middle. The *black rectangles* are the propagating depolarized zones (see Fig. 3.2a). **b** The skin surface with 16 equally spaced contacts covering the tendon to tendon distance. **c, d** Spatio-temporal representation of the 16 monopolar signals (**c**) and the 15 differential signals (**d**). *A* AP, generation interval, *B* AP propagation interval, *C* AP extinction interval

Since the two dipoles are of opposite polarity and their fields partially cancel out, the disappearance of dipole $D_1$ will eliminate the cancellation of dipole $D_2$, whose field will solely and fully determine the skin potential distribution. Accordingly, at time instant $t_3$, the monopolar voltages detected by the electrodes near the end of the fiber change shape and increase in amplitude. As dipole $D_2$ (the only one left after $t_3$) progressively squeezes against the end of the fiber (Fig. 3.6g), the intensity of its field decreases. When the two poles of D2 overlap and cancel out, $D_2$ likewise disappears, no field is generated, the AP is extinguished, and all voltages on the skin go to zero. These events take place in 2–4 ms and generate a transient in the surface potentials. This transient is referred to as the "end-of-fiber effect" or "fiber-end-effect" and is due to the extinction of the AP at the end of the fiber. Of course, a fiber has two ends and therefore there are two such events. If the NMJ is in the middle of the fiber and the conduction velocity is the same in both directions, the two events are simultaneous. Otherwise, they take place at different times.

Indeed, a similar event takes place during tripole generation at the NMJ. This is partially depicted in Figs. 3.5a and 3.4b. However, this generation event is less evident and not as easily detected because the generation of one tripole compensates and cancels the effect of the generation of the other.

Figure 3.7 shows the generation, propagation, and extinction of a muscle fiber AP in space and time, as observed using monopolar or differential recordings. The signals are simulated using a computer model. The fiber, its NMJ, and the two propagating depolarized areas are shown in Fig. 3.7a (for simplicity, the tripoles are not shown), and the surface of the skin and the array of detectors (electrodes) in Fig. 3.7b. The amplifiers are not illustrated, for reasons of simplicity. Note that the fiber is parallel to the skin surface and to the electrode array. Figure 3.7c shows the monopolar signals detected by each electrode with respect to a remote reference assumed to be at zero potential. The fiber is about 15 cm long and there are 16 electrodes equally spaced, with an inter-electrode distance of 1 cm.

The NMJ is in the middle, under electrode 8. In Fig. 3.7c, d, the dashed rectangle A shows the AP generation transient, the interval B the AP propagation, and the rectangle C the upper and lower end-of-fiber events, which are simultaneous because the fiber is innervated in the middle. Note that, because of the end-of fiber-effect, monopolar channels 1 and 2 show similar non-propagating signals and the same happens for channels 15 and 16. These signals are generated by the shrinking of the tripole (disappearance of D1) and its reduction to a dipole that shrinks further. As a result of the similarity of the monopolar signals, the corresponding differential signals will be small. The end-of-fiber effect is therefore much more evident in the monopolar than in the differential detection mode.

Note that monopolar channel 8 is quite different from its neighbors 7 and 9, such that the corresponding differential channels are large. The reader is invited to re-draw the signals for the case in which the NMJ is exactly centered between two electrodes.

Also note that the differential channels show propagating components that are narrower and sharper than in the monopolar case. This property would be enhanced by a further differentiation and computation of the double differential signals (see Sect. 2.7). The reader is invited to draw a third column of 14 signals, obtained by taking the difference between adjacent differential channels, and to comment on the result. Finally, notice the two-dimensional representation (2D) of the AP in time (horizontal axis) and space (vertical axis) shown in Fig. 3.7c, d.

Practically speaking, the AP of a single muscle fiber cannot be recorded because muscle fibers are activated in groups called "motor units". However, computer-simulated multichannel (linear array) APs are of great importance, not only as basic building blocks for motor unit and muscle models but also as tools that allow us to make interesting and important observations as well as to ask, and answer, questions that are relevant for understanding the EMG signals, such as:

Which signal set (monopolar, differential, or double differential) is the most suitable to identify the location of the NMJ of a muscle fiber?

Which signal set (monopolar, differential, or double differential) is the most suitable to study the end-of-fiber phenomenon?

Which signal set (monopolar, differential, or double differential) is the most suitable to estimate the velocity of propagation of the muscle fiber AP?

What would the signals in Fig. 3.7 look like if the fiber was not parallel to the skin but inclined with a given angle, such as in case of pinnate muscles?

What would the signals in Fig. 3.7 look like if the fiber had the NMJ near the end instead of in the middle?

What would a differential signal look like if taken between electrodes 7 and 9, or between 6 and 10, or between 5 and 11, in Fig. 3.7c? Could such signals be recovered if only differential signals (no monopolar) had been recorded?

Can the fiber length be estimated from the signals depicted in Fig. 3.7? Which set of signals would provide a better estimate?

## 3.5 The Motor Unit Action Potential (MUAP)

A muscle is made up of many motor units, with each motor unit (MU) consisting of a motor neuron and the group of muscle fibers it innervates. The fibers of a MU are therefore activated together. A single MU activation is indicated as a "discharge" or "firing" and it generates a "motor unit action potential" (MUAP), which is the sum of the contributions provided by the individual fibers that make up the MU. Figure 3.8 provides a description of a very simple MU, with only three fibers (*a*, *b*, and *c*).

The NMJs of the fibers of a MU are usually grouped in a narrow region described as the "innervation zone" (IZ), which is often (but not always) in the central part of the MU, as indicated in Fig. 3.8. In this example, an array of 16 electrodes, spaced 1 cm apart, is placed on the skin over the MU, whose fibers are parallel to the skin. The NMJ of fiber *a* is between electrode 8 and 9, that of fiber *b* under electrode 8, and that of fiber *c* under electrode 9. It is evident from the figure that the locations of the depolarized zones (tripoles) propagating upwards are not the same, relative to each other, as those of the depolarized zones propagating downwards. For example, the upwards tripole of fiber *b* is ahead of the others but the downwards tripole of the same fiber is behind the others. Consequently, the differential signals at the same distance from the IZ, above and below it, will not be identical and mirror-like, as in the case of a single fiber (Fig. 3.7d). In addition, the tripole generation transients of fibers *a*, *b*, and *c* will take place in different locations within the IZ and there-

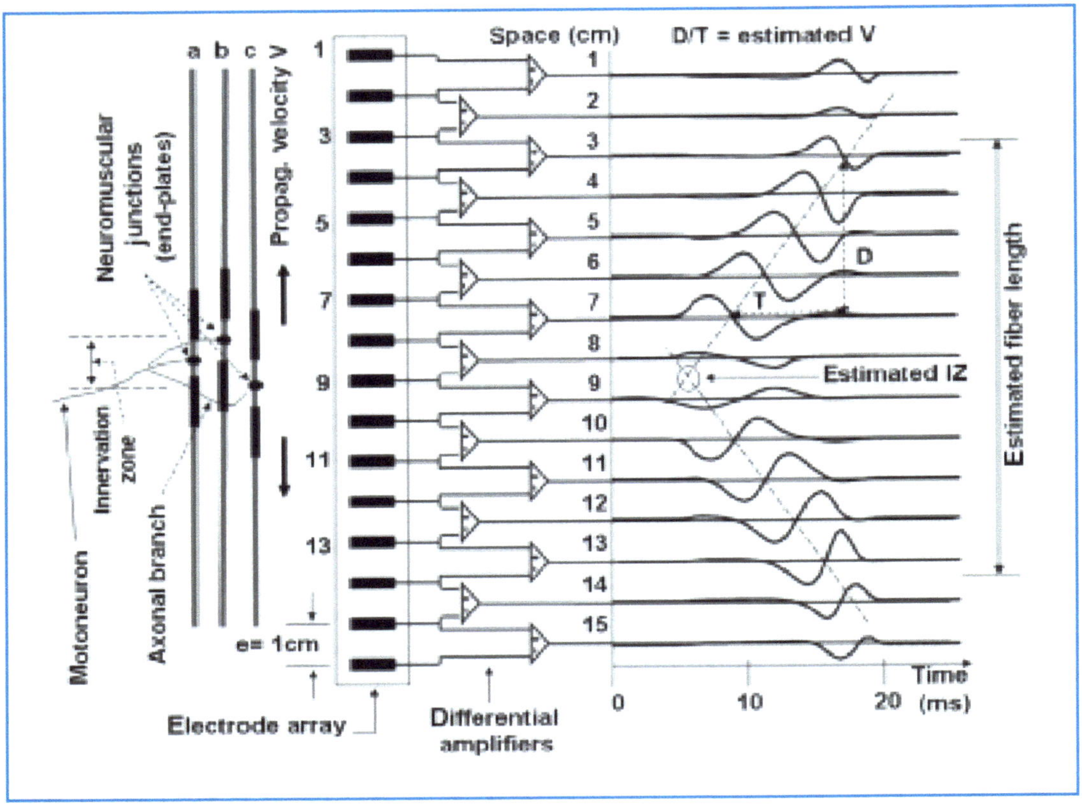


**Fig. 3.8** Example of a computer-generated motor unit action potential (MUAP) produced by a motor unit of three fibers (*a*, *b*, *c*). The MUAP is detected in differential mode from an array of 16 electrodes with an inter-electrode distance of 1 cm. Information concerning the innervation zone, fiber length, and conduction velocity of the MUAP can be obtained from the 15 signals. See text for further information

fore will have different effects on the differential channels 7–10 (electrodes 6–11), but also on the others, albeit to a lesser extent.

A considerable amount of information can be obtained from the signals depicted in Fig. 3.8, as reported in many publications (Merletti et al. 1999, 2001, 2003, among others). For example, the location of the IZ is evidently, by visual inspection, under electrode 9. A more accurate estimate can be obtained, using visual techniques, by drawing a line through the zero crossings of the propagating differential signals (avoiding those affected by the fiber-end-effect). If this is done on both sides of the IZ, the point where the two lines cross is a good estimate of the location of the center of the IZ. These lines can be drawn through the maxima or the minima of the differential signals with similar results.

The length of the fibers making up the MU can be roughly estimated as indicated in Fig. 3.8. Not all the fibers end in the same place. Thus, the transition from propagating to non-propagating signals due to the end-of-fiber effect may not be so distinct, such that the estimate is less accurate.

Conduction velocity may be visually estimated as the ratio between the distance D and the time interval T, as shown in Fig. 3.8 (where the conduction velocity is indicated with the symbol V). Again, also for this estimate, the channels affected by the end-of-fiber effect should not be considered. Estimation of the conduction velocity of a MU from a single firing is relatively simple but is considerably more complex for an interferential signal that is the sum of the contributions of many MUs, as discussed in the literature (Farina and Merletti, 2000, 2004).

## 3.6 The Interferential EMG Signal and the Issue of Electrode Location

Figure 3.9 shows 15 differential signals during a 250-ms epoch recorded, with a 16-electrode array, from a contracting biceps brachii muscle at 50% of the maximal voluntary force. More than a dozen MUAPs can be identified in this recording and a number of observations can be made:

1. All the MUAPs are generated by MUs that are all innervated under electrodes 7–8 (channel 7). The muscle presents only one IZ.
2. All the MUs terminate distally under electrodes 14, 15, 16 (channels 14, 15).
3. Most MUs terminate proximally under electrodes 1–2 (channel 1).
4. The MUs have about the same length (12–13 cm).
5. Some MUAPs are much larger than others, corresponding to MUs that are larger or more superficial than others.
6. Differences in conduction velocity between MUs cannot be estimated by eye (a computer with proper software is required) but all MUs have about the same conduction velocity.

The reader is invited to estimate the number of MUs that can be identified in this recording and to make additional observations concerning, for example, the channels that could be used for the estimation of muscle fiber conduction velocity. Figure 3.10 shows a similar recording from the biceps brachii of another subject. Here, the eight main MUAPs are identified and labeled. It can be seen that MUs 1, 3, 4, 5, and 8 are innervated un-

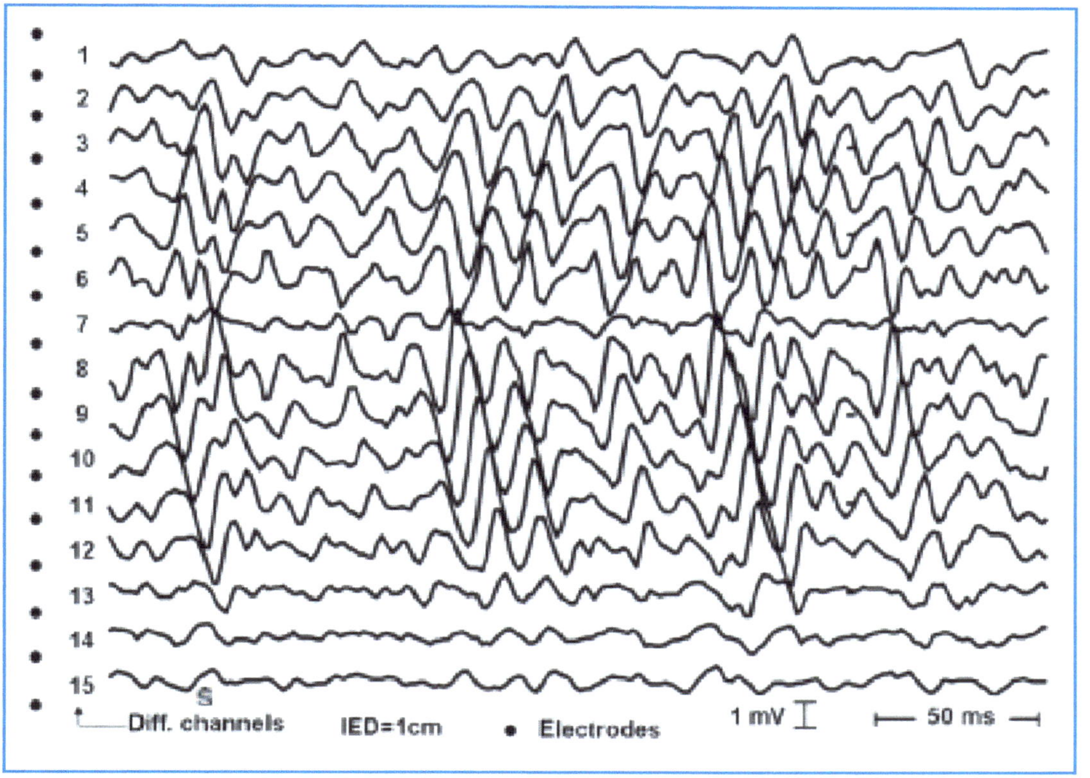


Fig. 3.9 Differential recording from a healthy biceps brachii contracting at about 50% of the maximal voluntary contraction. A linear array of 16 electrodes with an inter-electrode distance (IED) of 1 cm is applied in the (palpated) direction of the fibers. Several observations can be made by a visual analysis of the signals and concern the geometry and anatomy of the identifiable MU. See text for a discussion of these observations

der channel 7–8, and MUs 2, 6, and 7 under channel 10. Therefore, this muscle has two IZs: some MUs are innervated in one and some in the other. Only under channels 1–6 and 11–15 can we see unidirectional propagation. Some MUs are longer than the electrode array, some are shorter. The reader is invited to identify them and to consider the anatomy and geometry of the identifiable MUs. For example, are they all parallel to the skin and to the electrode array? Can repeated discharges of the same MUs be identified? How wide are the IZs?

As shown in Figs. 3.9 and 3.10, individual MU discharges (MUAPs) can be identified by eye and their most evident features estimated even without the use of computers. However, suitable computer programs provide more accurate global features (mean conduction velocity, localization of the one or two main IZs, global discharge rate). Other programs, now used for research only, can identify the repeating MUAPs of a single MU and the features of individual MUs. As shown in Figs. 3.10 and 3.11, 10–15 different MUAPs can be readily identified, corresponding to 10–15 MUs (the MUAPs are different). These MUs represent a small fraction of the many MUs activated in a human biceps brachii at about 50% of the maximal voluntary contraction (MVC).

The remaining MUs cannot be identified with current technology because they are too small or too deeply located. In either case, their MUAPs are too small to be reliably detected by the surface elec-

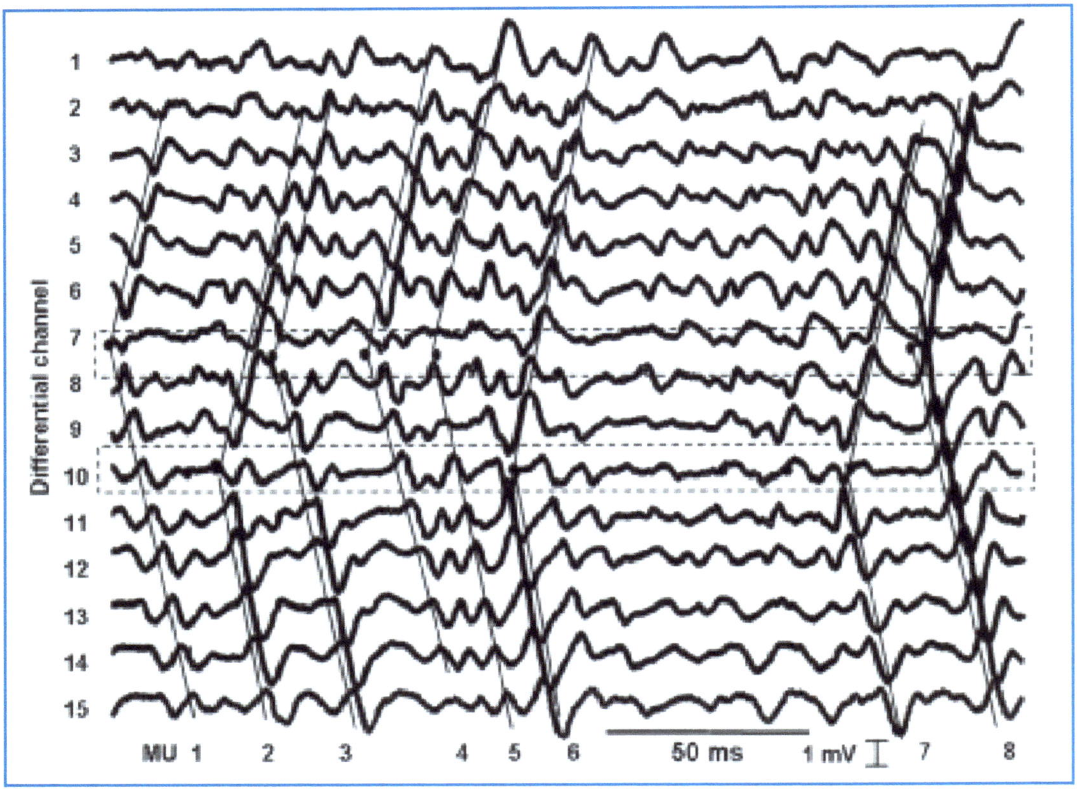


**Fig. 3.10** Differential recording from a healthy biceps brachii contracting at about 50% of the maximal voluntary contraction. A linear array of 16 electrodes with an inter-electrode distance (IED) of 1 cm is applied in the (palpated) direction of the fibers. Many observations can be made by a visual analysis of the signals and concern the geometry and anatomy of the identifiable MU. The eight MUs with the largest MUAPs are identified (by visual observation) and numbered. It can be seen that MUs 1, 3, 4, 5, and 8 are innervated under channel 7–8 while MUs 2, 6, and 7 are innervated under channel 10. The muscle has two regions of MU innervation. Some MUs are longer than the array. Visual observation does not show large differences in conduction velocity

trode system and cannot be separated from the background noise.

The differential EMG signal detected by a pair of electrodes applied on a muscle is the difference of the two monopolar signals (Figs. 2.5, 2.7). For example, the signal generated by a single fiber and detected between electrodes 2 and 6 in Fig. 3.7c is the difference between the two monopolar signals detected by these electrodes. Consider now electrodes 5 and 11 in Fig. 3.7c: they are symmetric with respect to the NMJ and their difference is zero (or very close to it, in case of minor asymmetries).

It can be demonstrated that the differential signal detected between any two electrodes (A and B) of a linear electrode array is the sum of the signals differentially detected by electrode pairs included between A and B. In the case of the previous single-fiber example (Fig. 3.7c), the same result may be obtained by adding the differential signals detected by the electrode pairs between the two chosen electrodes, as in Fig. 3.7d. In fact, assuming that the differences are taken in the top-down direction: $(V_5\text{-}V_6) + (V_6 - V_7) + (V_7 - V_8) + (V_8 - V_9) + (V_9 - V_{10}) + (V_{10} - V_{11}) = V_5 - V_{11}$ because all the other terms cancel out in the sum and what we obtain is the differential signal between $V_5$ and $V_{11}$. The same consideration applies in the case of a MU, with minor differences due to the fact that the NMJs of the fibers of the MU are scattered within the IZ and not aligned (see Fig. 3.8). Consequently, the sum of the differential signals between electrodes that are symmetric with respect to the estimated IZ will not be zero but will be small with respect to other channels.

Finally, consider, for example, in Fig. 3.9, the signals detected by channels 3 and 11. The differential signal $V_3 - V_{11}$ is the sum of the differential signals shown as channels 3–11. The sum is not really zero but very much smaller than the sum corresponding to other channel pairs. This is due to two reasons: (a) the fact that all the MUs are innervated in the same location (under channel 7) and (b) because the chosen electrode pair (3 and 11) is centered over the IZ (and therefore the two electrodes are equidistant from it).

Somewhat different is the situation depicted in Fig. 3.10, where two distinct IZs are clearly visible. Two electrodes centered over one IZ would not be centered over the other so that the MUs innervated in the first IZ would not provide a contribution whereas MUs innervated in the second IZ would provide a contribution to the differential signal detected by the two electrodes. In general, differential signals detected by an electrode pair centered over the IZ(s) of a muscle are smaller than those detected by an electrode pair placed over the propagation zone. This is one of the reasons for avoiding the IZ(s) of a muscle as the placement site of a single pair of electrodes. Optimal electrode placement is between the IZ(s) and one of the tendon endings. Of course, this implies knowing where the IZs are, but this can be determined using an electrode array, a multichannel amplifier, and a display of the recorded signals, as in Figs. 3.9 and 3.10. The second best option is to rely on an atlas of the innervation zones of superficial muscles (suitable for sEMG investigation), as provided in Part II of this book. Other considerations concern the location of the electrodes and the inter-electrode distance, particularly in the case of dynamic contractions. These issues have been extensively discussed in the literature for over 25 years (Masuda et al., 1985; Jensen et al., 1993; Farina et al., 2002; Rainoldi et al., 2004; Martin and Mac Isaac, 2006; Nishihara et al., 2008; Piitulainen et al., 2009a, b; Mesin et al., 2009a, among many others).

If the muscle contraction is not isometric, the muscle will shorten and the location of the IZ(s) will shift under the electrode array. This happens, to a more limited degree, even in the case of "isometric" contraction because of the elasticity of the tendons, which become slightly longer while the muscle becomes shorter (Martin and Mac Isaac, 2006; Piitulainen et al., 2009a, b).

In dynamic contractions, the phenomenon is much more evident and important because the IZ may shift under the electrode pair and cause a decrease in EMG amplitude that may be misinterpreted by the operator as a decrement of muscle activity rather than as a purely geometric phenomenon. This event is described in Fig. 3.11 for a single MU identified in the EMG of a healthy biceps brachii during flexion of the elbow from almost full extension to almost full flexion (100° change in the elbow's angle). Figure 3.11a depicts the MUAP of

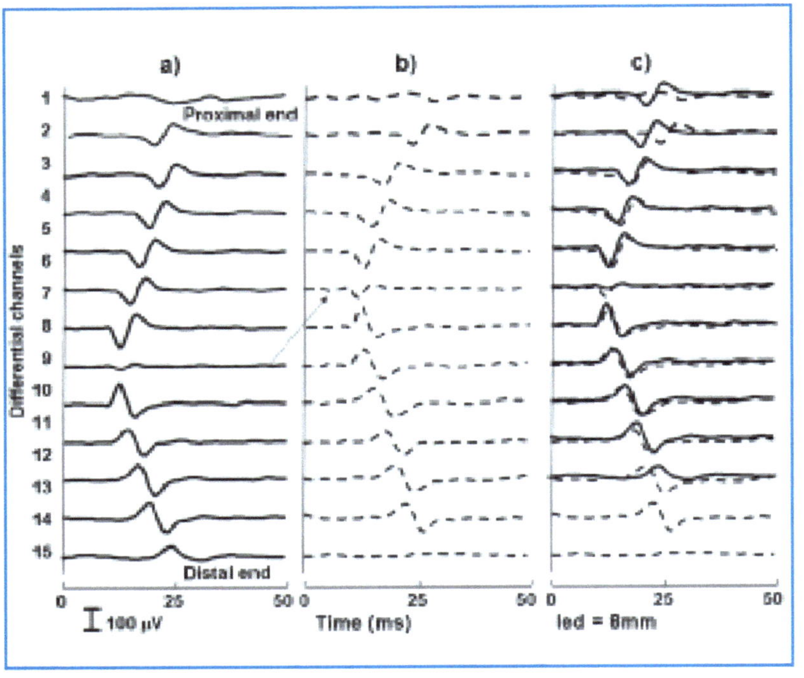


**Fig. 3.11 a** MUAP isolated from a healthy biceps brachii muscle during contraction and flexion of the elbow. The MUAP is detected with the elbow extended and tracked during slow flexion. **b** MUAP generated by the same MU after a 100° flexion of the elbow. A shift up of the innervation zone (IZ) is evident and indicates muscle shortening. **c** The MUAP indicated in **a** is shifted up by two inter-electrode distances (16 mm) and superimposed with that indicated in **b**, showing a good match of the channels near the IZ and suggesting that we are observing two MUAPs of the same MU at two lengths

the selected MU in the extended elbow position, and Fig. 3.11b the MUAP of the selected MU in the flexed elbow position. A shift of the innervation zone from channel 9 to channel 7 is evident and is about 16 mm (arrow in Fig. 3.11a, b). The MUAP shown in Fig. 3.11b is generated by the same MU as in Fig. 3.11a (it was tracked during slow elbow motion). However, the two MUAPs cannot be properly compared by shifting one with respect to the other and seeing if they match. This is because the muscle does not shift but instead shortens; therefore its proximal portion moves very little, the mid portion (the site of the IZ) moves more, and the distal portion much more. As a first rough approximation, for simplicity, we shift (rather than compress, as should be done) the signals up by 16 mm (two inter-electrode distances) and expect that at least the channels near the IZ will match. This is indeed what is shown in Fig. 3.11c, where the MUAP drawn with a solid line is shifted up by two channels and superimposed with the MUAP drawn with a dashed line. The mismatches in channels 1 and 2 and in channels 12 and 13 are due to the approximation implicit in the shifting.

Note that shortening of the muscle seems to appear as a signal decrease under channel 7 and a signal increase under channel 9. The same would happen in the case of the interferential signal (many MUs) for a muscle with a single IZ and, to a lesser degree, in a muscle with two or three IZs. *These changes, if observed using only one pair of electrodes, may be easily misinterpreted as an increase or a decrease of muscle activity, whereas they are due only to a change in the geometry of the system.* To further clarify this point, Fig. 3.12 shows 3 s of interferential EMG simultaneously detected from three electrode pairs placed over a healthy contracted biceps brachii. The pair shown in light gray is centered over the region of muscle innervation while the gray pair is next to it, and the black pair is in between the IZ and a tendon ending. It is evident that the amplitude of the signal depends on the electrode location. If the muscle shortens, the IZ will move upward and the two gray signals will increase; the black signal will be more affected by the end-of-fiber effect. Consequently, in dynamic contractions this geometric effect introduces serious limitations to the use of a single electrode pair, especially in muscles that are short and characterized by multiple IZs.

It should now be clear that even in muscles that are long and with fibers parallel to the skin (such as

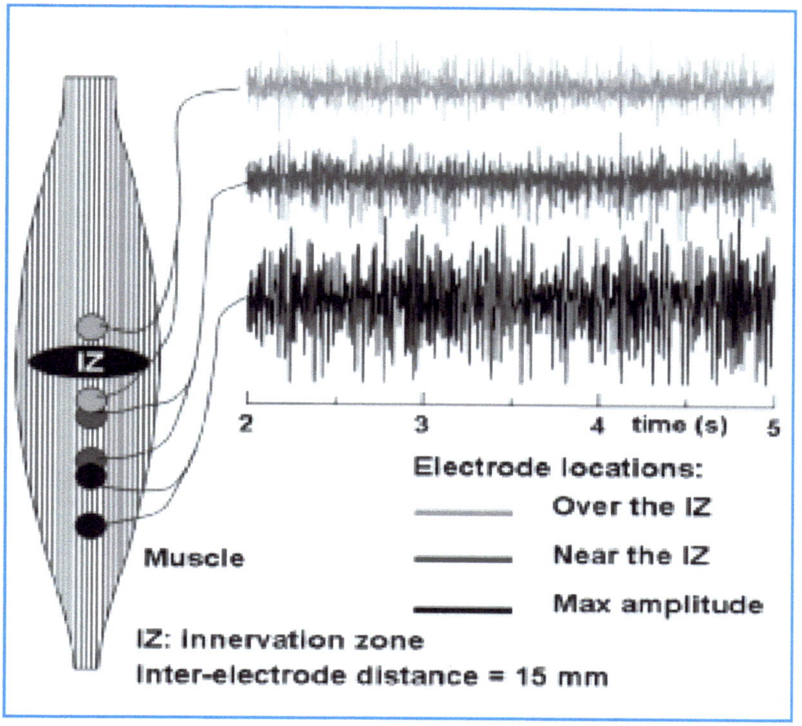


**Fig. 3.12** EMG readings from a healthy contracted biceps brachii using three electrode pairs with different locations with respect to the IZ and an inter-electrode distance of 15 mm. The light gray pair is over the IZ, the gray pair is next to it, and the black pair is in between the IZ and the tendon junction. A movement of the muscle under the electrodes would change the amplitude of the signals even if muscle activity does not change. This could lead to a misinterpretation of this purely geometric phenomenon and cause the operator to believe that muscle activity is increased or decreased

the biceps and the trapezius), a single electrode pair must be correctly placed, especially if the muscle has a single IZ (as in Fig. 3.9). The region of proper electrode location may be small and critical and the inter-electrode distance must be small. A small inter-electrode distance (< 15 mm) must be selected also for other reasons, discussed in Chapter 4. The use of electrode arrays provides insight into the geometric changes of a muscle that cannot be obtained using a single electrode pair. The situation is more complex in pinnate muscles, whose fibers are connected to an aponeurosis and are not parallel to the skin.

## 3.7 Muscle Architecture and sEMG: Pinnate Muscles

Many skeletal muscles are pinnate, that is, their fibers are not parallel to the skin but connect two tendon layers (aponeurosis), one superficial and one deep. The medial and lateral gastrocnemius and the biceps femoris are pinnate muscles. The sEMG potential generated on the skin above such muscles is very different from that generated by muscles with fibers parallel to the skin. Figure 3.13 shows this type of fiber arrangements and schematically depicts four MUs. The inset describes one of the fibers, its NMJ, and the two depolarized regions d1 and d2. Region d2 propagates downwards and deeper and its contribution to the surface potential distribution is very small whereas region d1 propagates upwards and its contribution to the surface potential increases as the source moves along the fiber, approaching the skin. In particular, extinction of the AP near the surface of the skin provides a large and non-propagating contribution to the surface potential distribution. When motor neuron A discharges, fibers 1, 2, 3, and 5 are activated and their end-of-fiber potentials appear under surface electrodes c–g in area A. When motor neuron B discharges, fibers 4, 6, 7, 8, and 10 are activated and their end-of-fiber potentials appear under surface electrodes d–i in area B. When motor neuron C discharges, fibers 9, 11, 12, and 13 are activated and their end-of-fiber potentials appear under surface electrodes h–n in area C. When motor neuron D discharges, fibers 12, 14,

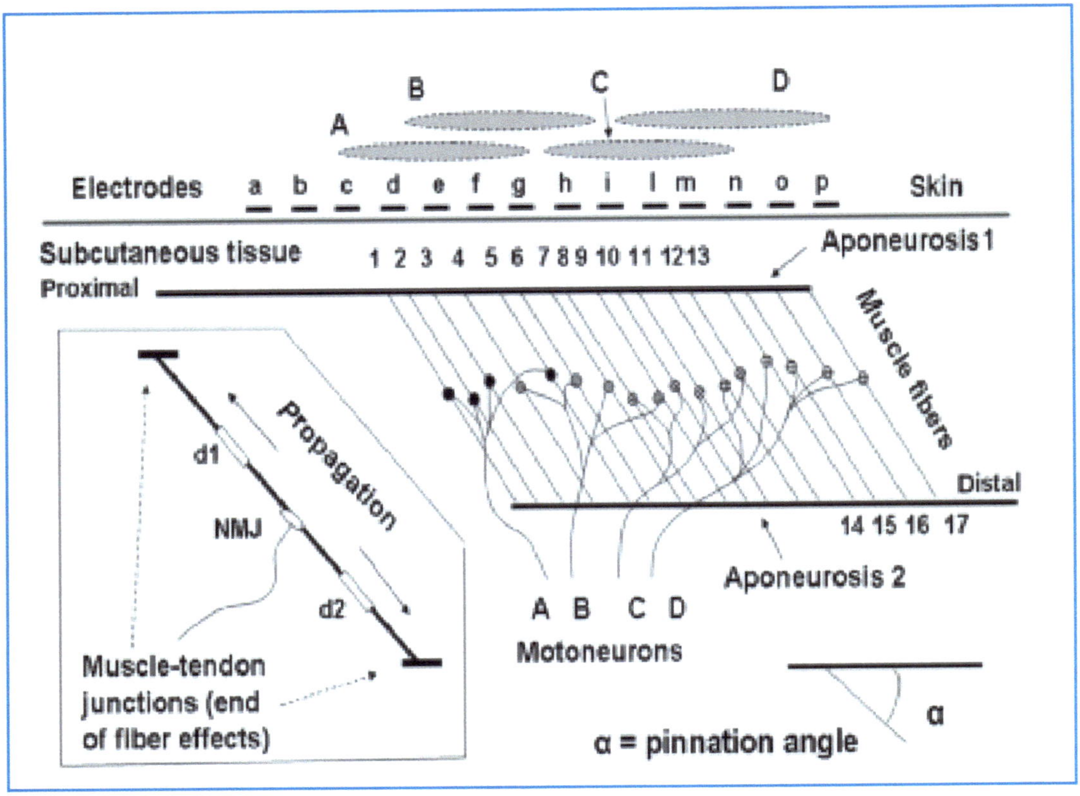


**Fig. 3.13** Structure of a pinnate muscle and location of the EMG potential distributions generated by the activation of different MUs. MU A generates potentials in region A, under electrodes c–g. MU B generates potentials in region B, under electrodes d–i, and so on. IZs and the propagations of APs are not detectable on the skin surface

15, and 17 are activated and their end-of-fiber potentials appear on the skin under surface electrodes i–p in area D.

Since MUs are activated asynchronously, subsequent maps of instantaneous surface potentials will appear above the gastrocnemius as a sequence of flashes momentarily activated in different regions above the muscle. Accordingly, the propagation of APs, as described in Figs. 3.9 and 3.10, cannot be observed in this muscle except in some cases in the vicinity of its distal end.

The EMG potential distributions present on the skin surface above the gastrocnemius muscle are mostly due to the end-of-fiber effect (see Figs. 3.6 and 3.7 in Sect. 3.4). Figure 3.13 suggests that the spatial support of the potential generated by each MU is correlated with the MU territory. In other words, MUs with a compact territory will produce distributions of surface potentials with a spatial extension smaller than that associated with MUs with a more widespread territory. Figure 3.14 shows a multichannel MUAP of a MU of a human gastrocnemius muscle obtained from a linear electrode array. The amplitude distribution of the individual channels along the array suggests a spatial distribution of fibers such as that schematically indicated in the left panel (Vieira et al., 2011).

In conclusion, the EMG potential distribution generated on the skin by a pinnate muscle is very different from that of a muscle with fibers parallel to the skin. This difference is greater when the pinnation angle is greater; however, even small angles (5–10°) make the signal substantially different from the one generated by MUs with fibers parallel to the skin. For the reasons indicated above, in general, muscle fiber conduction velocity cannot be reliably estimated from a pinnate muscle. However, the distal part of the gastrocnemius often al-

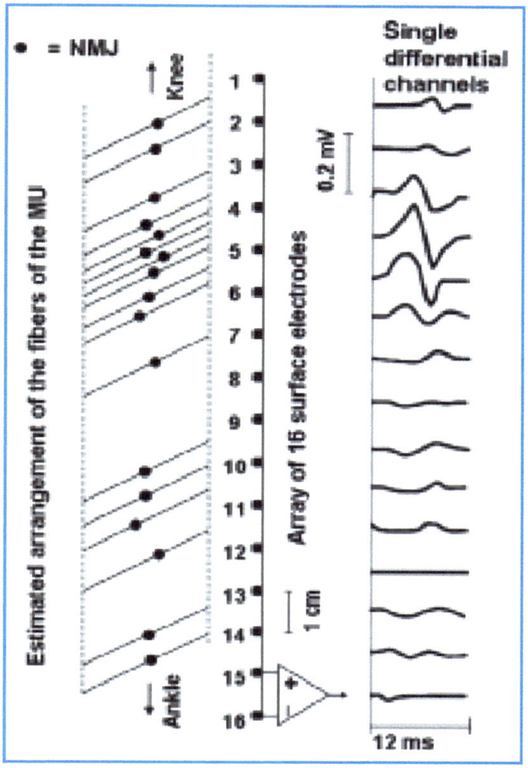


Fig. 3.14 Single differential potential distribution of a MU discharge and an array of 16 equally spaced electrodes placed on the skin above the medial gastrocnemius muscle. The estimated arrangement of the fibers of the activated MU, that is compatible with the signals depicted in the right panel, is shown. The *black dots* represent a possible arrangement of the NMJ of the individual fibers of the MU. The superficial differential potentials are approximately aligned in time, represent mostly end-of-fiber effects, and do not show propagation. The *vertical dotted lines* are the two aponeuroses of the muscle

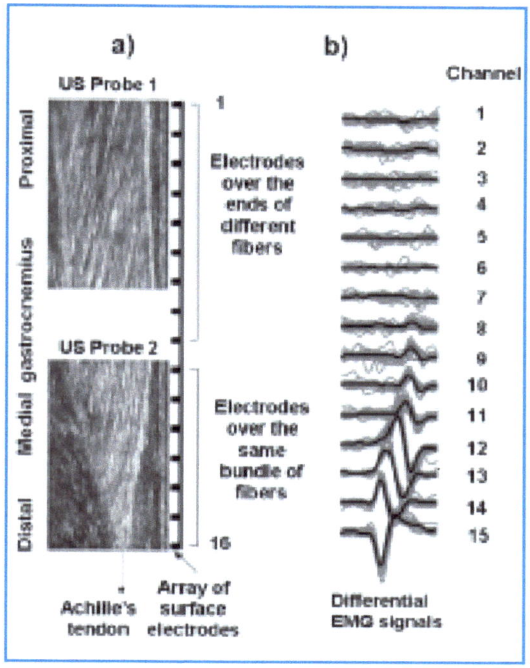


Fig. 3.15 a Two echographic sections of a medial gastrocnemius muscle obtained from two ultrasound probes, one more proximal and the other near the Achille's tendon. b Single differential potential distributions of multiple discharges of a MU are depicted with superimposed gray lines. Their average is depicted in black. Note that the MU is distal and has a very narrow IZ under electrode 15. The AP of the MU propagates in the distal to proximal direction, from electrode 15 to electrodes 10–11. The fibers of this MU attach to the superficial aponeurosis under electrodes 10–11. In this case, the IZ and AP propagation can be detected by the surface electrode array. However, the estimate of conduction velocity is incorrect because the fibers are not parallel to the skin. (Reproduced from Fig. 8 of Vieira et al. 2011)

lows such estimates because, in this region, some electrodes of an array may be above the same bundle of fibers such that the propagating potentials are detectable. The pinnation angle would of course bias the estimate of conduction velocity. Figure 3.15a provides an example, as depicted by two ultrasonographic images of a medial gastrocnemius (one more proximal and one more distal). Figure 3.15b shows repeated MUAPs of the same MU and their average template. The IZ of the depicted MU is narrow and under electrodes 14–15 (Vieira et al., 2011).

## Suggested Reading

Farina D, Merletti R (2000) Comparison of algorithms for estimation of EMG variables during voluntary isometric contractions. J Electromyogr Kines 10:337-49

Farina D, Merletti R (2004) Methods for estimating muscle fibre conduction velocity from surface electromyographic signals. Med Biol Eng Comput 42:432-445

Farina D, Cescon C, Merletti R (2002) Influence of anatomical, physical, and detection-system parameters on surface EMG. Biol Cybern. 86:445-56

Jensen C, Vasseljen O, Westgaard RH (1993) The influence of electrode position on bipolar surface electromyogram recordings of the upper trapezius muscle. Eur J Appl Physiol 67:266-73

Martin S, Mac Isaac D (2006) Innervation zone shift with changes with joint angle in the brachial biceps. J Electromyogr Kinesiol 16:144-148

Masuda T, Miyano H, Sadoyama T (1985) The position of innervation zones in the biceps brachii investigated by surface electromyography. IEEE Trans on Biomed Eng 32:36-42

Merletti R, Farina D, Granata A (1999) Non-invasive assessment of motor unit properties with linear electrode arrays. Electroencephalogr Clin Neurophysiol 50:293-300

Merletti R, Rainoldi A, Farina D (2001) Surface electromyography for non-invasive characterization of muscles. Exerc Sport Sci Rev 29:20-25

Merletti R, Farina D, Gazzoni M (2003) The linear electrode array: a useful tool with many applications. J Electromyogr Kinesiol 13:37-47

Mesin L, Merletti R, Rainoldi A (2009) Surface EMG: the issue of electrode location. J Electromyogr Kinesiol 19:719-26

Nishihara K, Kawai H, Gomi T et al (2008) Investigation of optimum electrode locations by using automated surface electromyography analysis technique. IEEE Trans Biomed Eng 55:636-642

Piitulainen H, Bottas R, Linnamo V et al (2009a) Effect of electrode location on surface electromyography changes due to eccentric elbow flexor exercise. Muscle Nerve 40:617-25

Piitulainen H, Rantalainen T, Linnamo V et al (2009b) Innervation zone shift at different levels of isometric contraction in the biceps brachii muscle. J Electromyogr Kinesiol 19:667-75

Rainoldi A, Melchiorri G, Caruso I (2004) A method for positioning electrodes during surface EMG recordings in lower limb muscles. J Neurosci Meth 134:37-43

Vieira TMM, Loram ID, Muceli S et al (2011) Postural activation of the human medial gastrocnemius muscle: how large is the territory of motor units? J Physiol 15:589(Pt 2):431-443

# EMG Imaging: Geometry and Anatomy of the Electrode-Muscle System

4

**Abstract**

EMG imaging is the focus of this chapter. The concepts of instantaneous two-dimensional potential distribution and image interpolation are discussed with respect to sEMG potential maps generated by fusiform or pinnate muscles. Sequences of images forming "movies" that reflect the generation and propagation of motor unit action potentials, as well as anatomical information concerning the location of the innervation zone, are annotated in order to illustrate how the underlying muscle anatomy and physiology can be unveiled by suitable processing of the sEMG collected with a 2D array of electrodes.

## 4.1 The Concept of Sampling and Interpolation of One-Dimensional Signals

Bioelectric signals (such as EMG) are analog; that is, they are continuous and smooth and do not change abruptly in space or in time. So are the signals in space depicted in Fig. 2.9 (dotted lines) or those in time depicted in Fig. 2.10 (solid lines). Digital computers, however, accept only numbers (digits) at their input. Therefore, an analog signal varying in space or in time must be converted into a sequence of numbers. This operation is performed in two steps: (1) sampling and (2) analog to digital conversion (A/D conversion). The underlying concepts of these two operations are illustrated below.

To "sample" a signal means to take "samples" from it. The samples are usually equally spaced along the x axis (space or time). Consider the smooth signal segment represented by a dashed line in Fig. 4.1a. Six equally spaced samples ($S_1$–$S_6$) are taken from it and their values are represented by the lengths of the vertical thin lines. In computer memory, the signal represented by the dashed line does not exist; only the sampled values. The more samples we take per unit time (or space), the better we can represent the original signal, i.e., the "resolution" will be greater; however, a larger computer file will be needed to store the acquired information. A signal must be sampled above a minimal rate, which depends on how fast the signal is changing (see Chapter 5). The sampling frequency is the number of samples taken per second (Samples/s or S/s). If the sampling frequency is above this minimal rate (referred to as the "Nyquist rate") the original signal can be reconstructed without error from its samples. Otherwise an error arises due to a phenomenon called "aliasing."

To convert a signal from analog to digital form requires that the value of each sample (the length of each vertical line in Fig. 4.1a) is transformed into a number that can be stored in a computer memory cell in binary format. After this operation has been performed, the original signal is represented by a sequence of numbers corresponding to the black dots of Fig. 4.1a. If we prefer a finer representation of the signal we could "interpolate" the stored numbers to increase the number of samples. Note that interpolation is an approximation and is *not equivalent* to a higher sampling frequency.

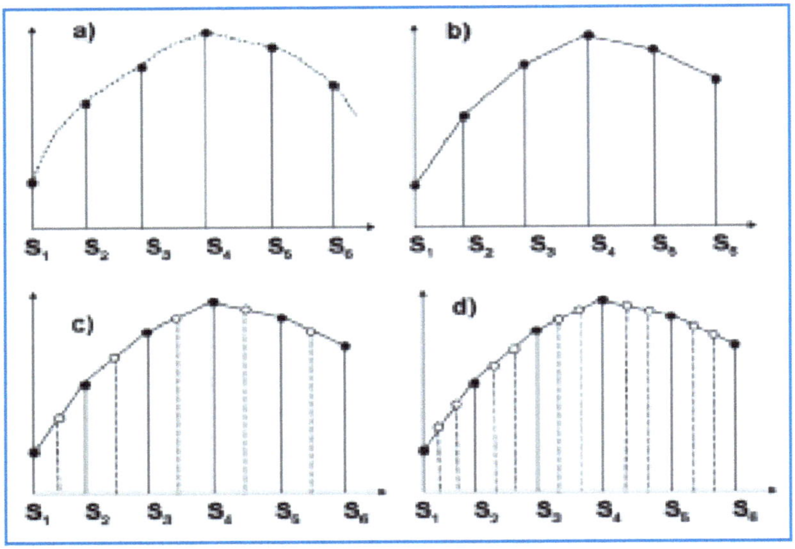


**Fig. 4.1** **a** Example of an analog signal sampled at time instants $S_1$–$S_6$. The sample values are indicated by *dots*. **b** The sample values are interconnected by straight segments. **c** The sampling frequency is artificially doubled by taking an "interpolated" sample in the middle of each segment. **d** The sampling frequency is artificially tripled by taking two "interpolated" samples within each segment. This process introduces approximations and is not equivalent to sampling at a higher rate

A very simple way to interpolate the stored samples is to imagine that they are interconnected by segments, as indicated in Fig. 4.1b, and to take one or more intermediate values between each pair of the original samples. The new artificial samples are indicated by the empty circles in Fig. 4.1c, d. This operation results in an approximation of the original signal, in a process is called "linear interpolation." However, there are other interpolation processes that may provide a better approximation of the original signal in that they use a curvilinear rather than a linear approximation.

## 4.2 The Concept of Sampling and Interpolation of Two-Dimensional Signals

The potential distribution on the surface of the skin, generated by a source moving below the skin, is the analog of a movie describing this potential, which evolves in space and time under a 2-dimensional array (see Fig. 2.11). Each "frame" of the movie is an image at a specific time instant and defines an area in the x and y directions. The individual frames are made up of pixels, defined by the electrodes, that we assume to be equally spaced in the x and y directions. The number of frames per second is the sampling frequency in time. Therefore, the EMG potential distribution is "sampled" in space by the electrodes and in time by the sampling frequency.

The number of pixels in space is limited by the number of electrodes and by their interelectrode distance (e.g., 64, 128, or more) such that interpolation in space may be needed to obtain an image smoother than that presented, for example, in Fig. 2.11b and reported again in Fig. 4.2b. Spatial interpolation is obtained with mathematical algorithms that estimate the values of the potential in between electrodes, as indicated in the example of Fig. 4.2c in the case of four pixels. The process is conceptually similar to that of interpolation in one dimension but the mathematical instruments to perform bidimensional interpolation are more complex.

## 4.3 Two-Dimensional EMG Detection in Fusiform Muscles

Figure 4.3 shows a single frame (that is, a single time sample or instantaneous picture) of a motor unit action potential (MUAP) distribution under an electrode grid with five columns and 13 rows (one electrode missing in one corner) and an 8-mm interelectrode distance. Since the instantaneous potential distribution shown in Fig. 4.3 is a "longitudinal single differential" (LSD), that is, the difference between the monopolar potentials of adjacent electrodes along each column (see Fig.

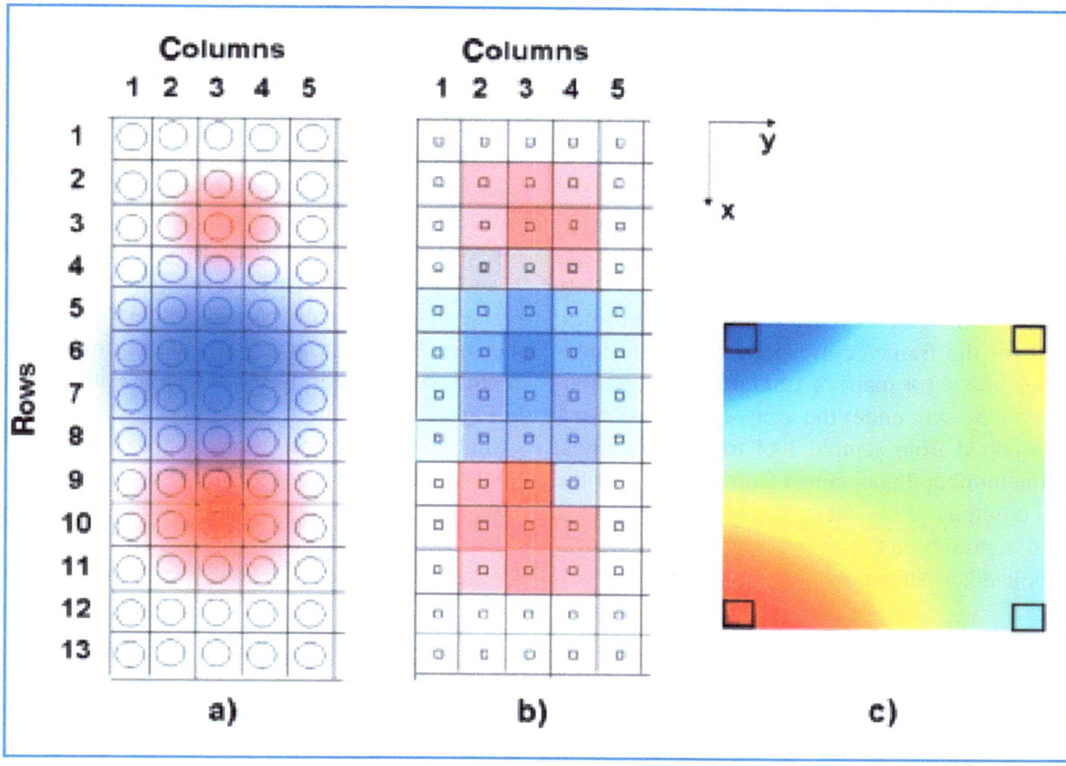


**Fig. 4.2** **a** Example of an instantaneous analog distribution of potential (*red* = positive, *blue* = negative, *white* = zero) under an electrode array (*circles*) defining the pixels of the detected image (*squares of the grid*). **b** Pixels of the image detected by the electrode grid. **c** Example of interpolation in two dimensions: four electrodes of four colors are shown (*small squares blue, red, yellow, and turquoise*); intermediate colors are defined by the interpolation in space performed between the pixels

2.9a, b), there will only be 12 EMG channels per column. Accordingly, in Fig. 4.3a the signal array comprises five columns and 12 rows and represents signals rather than electrodes (see Fig. 2.9b, where 15 LSD signals are generated by 16 electrodes). This array has an interelectrode distance of 8 mm and covers an area of 32 × 88 mm. The columns are aligned with the fiber direction. The innervation zone (IZ) of the motor unit (MU) is above the top of Fig. 4.3a and the potential propagates downwards, while the IZ of the MU is to the right of Fig. 4.3b and the potential propagates leftwards. The instantaneous LSD potential distribution under the array is interpolated in both the x and y directions in order to produce a smoother image. The potential values are represented by colors, with red indicating a positive potential, green a zero potential, and blue a negative potential. The array is placed over the biceps brachii, whose fibers are parallel to the skin.

Figure 4.3b presents the same information shown in Fig. 4.3a but in a different way. The LSD potential distribution is depicted in a third dimension (the amplitude axis) and as a color scale. Note that the grid of the surface representing the instantaneous potential distribution is finer than the grid of original channels (circles) because of the interpolation process. A sequence of images, like that in Fig. 4.3a, b, equally spaced in time, for example 0.5 ms apart, provides a movie describing the evolution in time of the 2D potential distribution under the array.

In Fig. 4.3 the electrode grid is placed on one side of the IZ. In Fig. 4.4a, the electrode grid of five columns and 13 rows is centered over the IZ and detects 5 × 12 LSD signals, depicted in Fig.

4.4b, each one vs. time, for a 30-ms interval. This interval is chosen to incorporate a MUAP and its propagation from the IZ to the two ends of the array. The 12 LSD signals detected from each of the five columns of the signal array are sampled in time at the frequency of 2000 S/s, that is every 0.5 ms. Six frames are selected, 2 ms apart from each other (that is one frame every four), and are labeled as frames 1, 2, 3, 4, 5, and 6 in Fig. 4.4b. They are indicated by the vertical dashed lines. Each of the frames corresponds to an instantaneous image (or map) of LSD potential distribution on the skin under the array. Frame number 1 is obtained from sample 1 of the five columns, frame number 2 is obtained from sample 2 of the five columns (2 ms later), etc. Each time sample (1–6) represents a frame or map in space that is interpolated, as shown in Fig. 4.4c.

Figures 3.4–3.7 in the previous chapter help us in understanding Fig. 4.4. Frame 1 shows the generation of a dipole at the IZ (under rows 6–7) as described in Fig. 3.4a. Frames 2 and 3 show the generation and separation of two tripoles moving, respectively, up and down the array, as described in Fig. 3.4c. Observe the top-down sequence of + – + – + regions, just like the left-right sequence of + – + – + regions depicted in Figs. 3.4c and 3.5d. Frames 4–6 show the separation of the tripoles and the formation of a zero potential region in the central part of the array, as seen in one dimension in Figs. 3.5d and 3.7.

In Fig. 4.4b, we can observe that the signals are stronger under columns 3 and 4, indicating that the motor unit whose action potential (AP) is being observed is under these two columns. The same conclusion can be reached by observing that the most

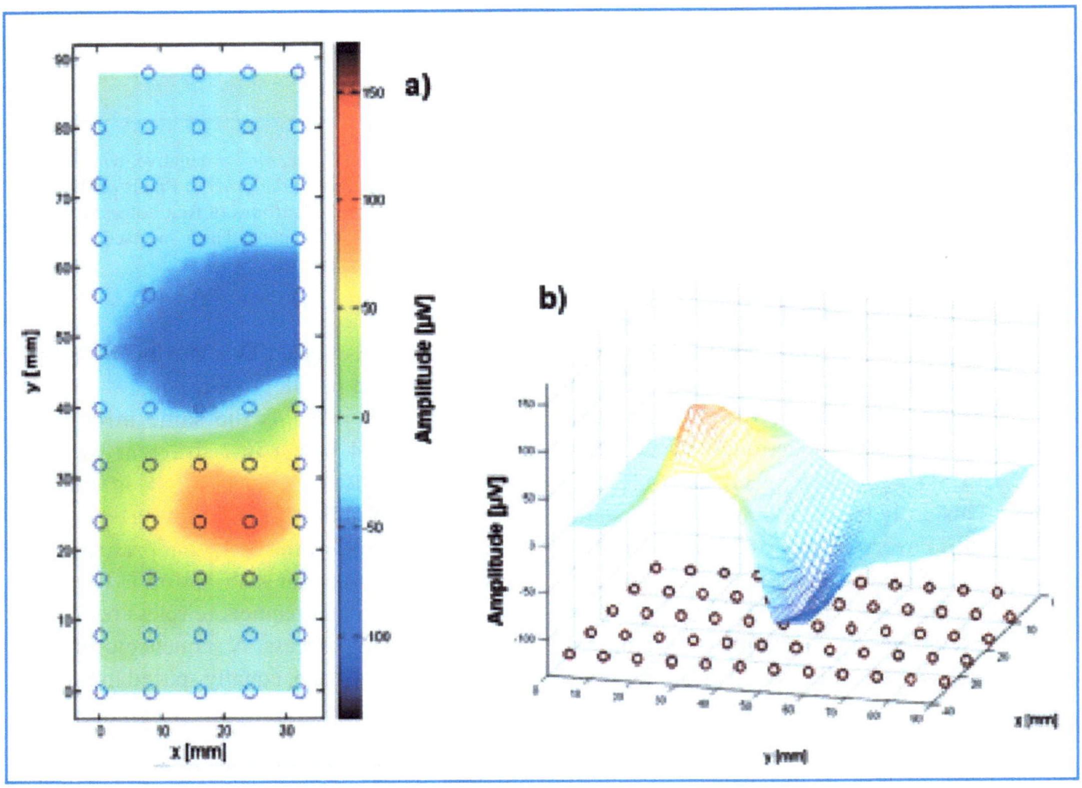


**Fig. 4.3** **a** Example of an electrode grid (*circles*) of five columns by 12 rows, with an 8-mm interelectrode distance, detecting a MUAP propagating downwards underneath the grid. The LSD potential distribution is represented by colors (see scale) and is interpolated. **b** The same potential distribution depicted in **a** is represented as a colored surface in three dimensions. Signals are detected from the biceps brachii muscle during a low-level isometric contraction (Courtesy of Dr. A. Holobar)

intense colors are in the rightmost portion of the frames in Fig. 4.4c, indeed under columns 3 and 4. The six dashed lines, numbered 1–6, depicted in Fig, 4.4b are 2 ms apart and represent the six frames depicted in Fig. 4.4c. To see this correspondence, consider all the dashed lines labeled as “1” in Fig. 4.4b. The dashed line “1” in column 1 identifies 12 samples (the first is missing) from column 1. The dashed line “1” in column 2 identifies 12 samples from column 2, and so on up to column 5. All these samples are taken at the same time and define a frame of 60 LSD values (12 × 5 pixels). The same applies to the dashed lines 2, 3, 4, 5, and 6.

Note that the grid depicted in Fig. 4.2 has 13 × 5 pixels (monopolar mode) that correspond to 12 × 5 pixels (LSD mode) in Fig. 4.4. See also Fig. 3.5, where the 16 monopolar channels generate 15 differential channels. The six frames, of 15 × 5 pixels each, are then interpolated in two dimensions (see Fig, 4.2c) to produce the six images of Fig. 4.4c. Finally, consider again Fig. 3.5. The propagating tripoles modeling the sources are mirror-like but the sequence of + and – inputs of the amplifiers is not mirror-like. This results in the propagating waves (sampled in space) collected at the 15 outputs of the differential amplifiers and showing a negative leading swing in the rightwards propagations and a positive leading swing in the leftwards propagations. Similarly, and for the same reason, the downwards propagation in Fig. 4.4c has a negative leading swing whereas the upwards propagation has a positive leading swing.

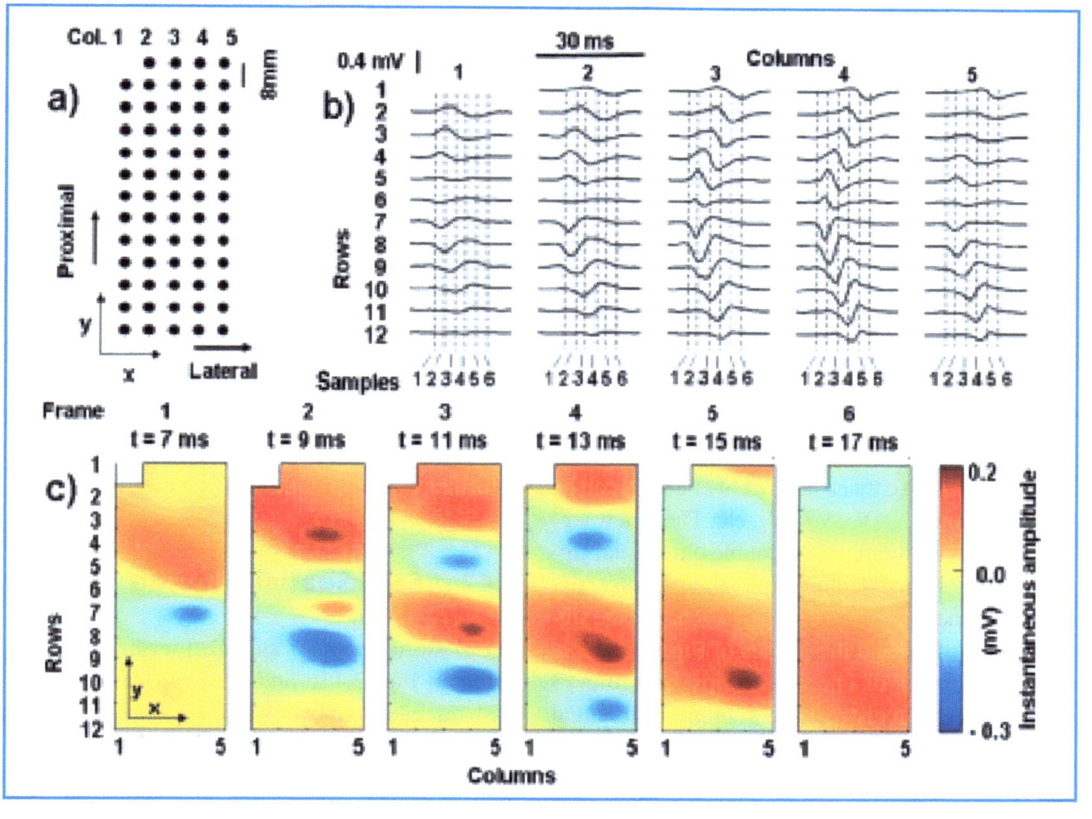


**Fig. 4.4** **a** Electrode grid (13 rows by five columns and one electrode missing in the top left corner). **b** Time course (over 30 ms) of the LSD signals detected along each column (columns 1–5, 12 channels per column). Observe the well-defined innervation zone under rows 6–7. The LSD signals are sampled at 2000 S/s (0.5 ms between samples) generating 2000 frames/s. Six time frames, 2 ms apart, are indicated by *vertical dashed lines*. **c** The six frames of the instantaneous LSD EMG amplitude are aligned from left to right and show the generation (under row 6–7) and propagation (upwards and downwards) of a MUAP. See text for additional explanations

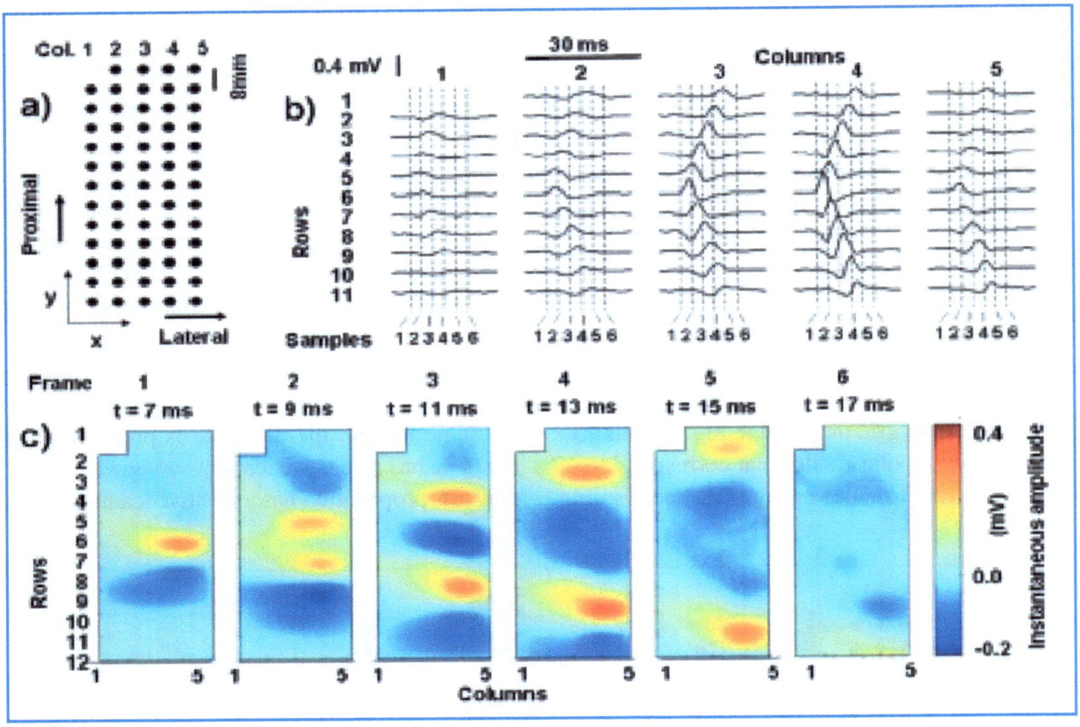


Fig. 4.5 a Electrode grid (13 rows by five columns and one electrode missing in the top left corner). b Time course (over 30 ms) of the LDD signals detected along each column (1–5, 11 channels per column). Each channel is the difference between two adjacent channels of the same column of Fig. 4.4. The LDD signals are sampled at 2000 S/s (0.5 ms between samples) generating 2000 frames/s. Six time frames, 2 ms apart, are indicated. c The six frames of the instantaneous LDD EMG amplitude are side by side from left to right. See text for additional explanations

Consider again Fig. 3.5 and the differential detection (LSD) that produces $V_1 = V_A - V_B$ and $V_2 = V_B - V_C$, etc. The process of longitudinal differentiation can be repeated so that a new set of channels can be obtained from $V_1 - V_2$, $V_2 - V_3$, etc. These new signals are called "longitudinal double differential signals" (LDD). This second differentiation in space is applied to the signals of Fig. 4.4b to generate the signals of Fig. 4.5b and the frames of Fig. 4.5c. Note that the number of channels drops from the 13 monopolar channels to the 12 single differential channels to the 11 double differential channels.

The images of Fig. 4.5c are "sharper" and more "focused," or less "blurred," than those of Fig. 4.4. The operation transforming the monopolar signals into the single differential signals (Figs. 3.5 and 3.7) implies the application of a spatial filter. The operation transforming the single differential signals of Fig. 4.4 into the double differential signals of Fig. 4.5 implies a second application of the same spatial filter to the output of the first. The concept of a spatial filter was already introduced in Fig. 2.11c and is further explored in the next section.

## 4.4 EMG Spatial Filtering

The basic concept of spatial filtering was illustrated in Fig. 2.11c and discussed in Sect. 2.8. With our additional knowledge we can now revisit this concept, applying it to 2D signals.

Monopolar detection provides the signal detected between each EMG electrode and a remote point taken as reference. Any algebraic combination of the signals detected in monopolar mode is referred to as a "spatial filtering" operation. For example, the averaging of the potentials detected by a sub-group of electrodes is a form of spatial filtering. Computing the difference between monopolar potentials detected by adjacent electrodes along each column of the array (see Fig. 3.5) is a spatial filtering operation, i.e., the longitudinal single differentiation discussed above, which generates a set of LSD signals. Computing a second difference between adjacent LSD channels along each column is a spatial filtering operation, the longitudinal double differentiation discussed above, which generates a set of LDD signals.

Single or double differential signals also can be computed transversally to the direction of the muscle fibers and are referred to as "transversal single differential" (TSD) or "transversal double differential" (TDD) signals. Many other filters can be designed to make the detection system more or less selective, with a smaller or larger detection volume.

Any spatial filtering operation implies advantages and disadvantages and is performed to achieve a specific objective. Some examples follow.

The single differential filter applied to electrode pairs, in a direction either parallel (LSD) or transversal (TSD) to the muscle fibers, removes signal components that are identical in all monopolar channels, such as most of the interference from power lines (50 Hz or 60 Hz, depending on the country). The LSD filter provides easy identification of the IZ (minimal amplitude and/or phase reversal of the signal, as shown in Figs. 3.7–3.9). In addition, the LSD signals provide information about the channels that should be selected for estimating muscle fiber conduction velocity (Fig. 3.8) and about the shift of the IZ during slow dynamic contractions (Fig. 3.11). However, some information available from monopolar signals is lost (the question: "which signals have a difference of x units at a given time?" has infinite answers) and the "end-of-fiber" effect (Figs. 3.6, 3.7) is strongly attenuated, which may or may not be desirable depending on the application. The LDD filter further reduces the power line interference and the end-of-fiber effect.

These components are non-propagating such that the multichannel estimate of conduction velocity is more correct. In addition, an LDD filter attenuates slow signals (which change slowly in space and are mostly due to far away sources) and provides a sharper image of nearby sources, as shown in Figs. 4.4 and 4.5. However the IZ is not easily detectable from this signal and three electrodes are required instead of two.

The smoothing of rapidly varying signals and the enhancement of signals slowly varying in space may be obtained by a "moving average" filter, such as by averaging four monopolar signals (2 × 2 electrodes) and by applying this process over the entire 2D array.

"Differentiating" filters enhance signal components that propagate along the electrode array and attenuate those that are common (that is, those simultaneously present with similar or identical amplitudes) across electrodes. This property is desirable to estimate the AP conduction velocity of muscle fibers in fusiform muscles with fibers parallel to the skin. However, interpretation is more difficult in cases of pinnate muscles (Figs. 3.13, 3.14), as the fibers are not parallel to the skin and the superficial signal is mostly due to the non-propagating end-of-fiber effect (see Figs. 3.6, 3.7). In this case, estimates of conduction velocity are incorrect.

## 4.5 The Issue of Interelectrode Distance and Electrode Location

An electrode array samples the surface potential distribution in space, as shown in Fig. 3.5b, d for a linear (1D) array and in Figs. 4.2b and 4.3 for a 2D electrode array (grid). If the electrodes are relatively far apart and an AP distribution (in space) is therefore described only by a few samples, it is impossible to reconstruct a spatial map of instantaneous potential. Interpolation processes (in space) provide, in this case, an incorrect distribution. Considerations deriving from signal processing theory indicate that the interelectrode distance should be in the range of 4–10 mm to provide at least a few samples for each MU potential (see Fig. 3.5b, d). Large interelectrode distances and improper electrode locations may lead to very misleading results.

Consider the muscle fiber depicted in Fig. 3.5c, innervated under electrode I of a linear array. Figure 4.6b–e shows the spatial distribution of the monopolar signals at four time instants ($t_1$–$t_4$) after separation of the two tripoles traveling in op-

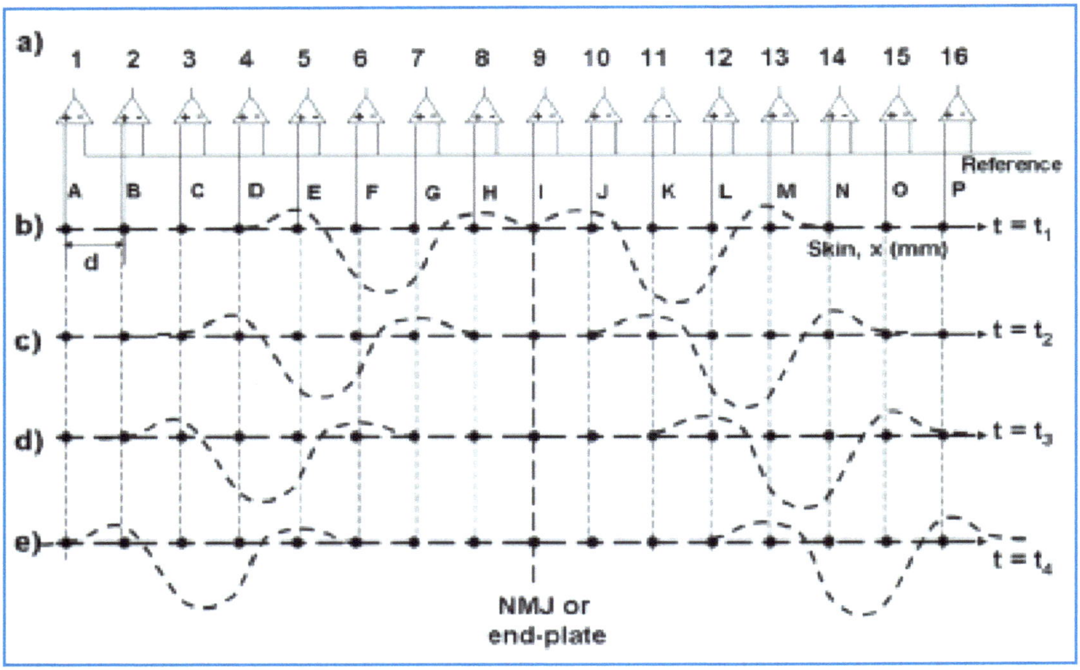


**Fig. 4.6** **a** Linear array of amplifiers detecting monopolar signals generated by a single fiber, parallel to the skin, whose NMJ is under electrode I. **b** Monopolar potential distribution under the electrodes at time t1 after a discharge of the fiber, when the two tripoles have just separated. **c–e** Same as in b at subsequent time instants t2, t3, t4 as the two tripoles move, respectively, to the right and left of the NMJ. Observe that any pair of electrodes placed symmetrically with respect to the NMJ (electrode I) provide the same monopolar potential and therefore a zero differential potential at any time. See also Figs. 3.5, 3.7 and 3.8. In practice, a small signal is provided due to noise and small asymmetries

posite directions. Single differential signals detected between electrode pairs that are symmetric with respect to electrode I (such as electrodes H and J, or G and K, etc.) would all be zero at all times, because they are the differences between equal monopolar voltages. In this case, a MU (or an entire muscle) whose fibers are all innervated under electrode I would not produce any differential voltage between two electrodes placed symmetrically with respect to that electrode.

In real conditions, the neuromuscular junctions (NMJs) of the fibers of a MU are scattered in the IZ, as indicated in Fig. 3.8, and all the MUs of a muscle may be innervated in the same location (as in Fig. 3.9) or in slightly different locations (as in Fig. 3.10). In either case, one electrode pair with interelectrode distance of 15–20 mm centered over the IZ of a MU would not correctly detect the differential signals from that MU. Similarly, one pair of nearby electrodes centered over the IZ of a muscle would detect a small, noisy, and non-representative differential signal from the muscle.

This issue was discussed in Sect. 3.6 and can now be considered with respect to a 2D potential detection. The above issues have been extensively presented in the literature over the last 20 years and European recommendations have been developed (Hermens et al. 2000; Jensen et al. 1993; Rau and Disselhorst-Klug 1997; Disselhorst-Klug et al. 1997; Mesin et al. 2009; De Nooij 2009; Martin and Mac Isaac 2006; Merletti et al. 2008).

## 4.6 Two-Dimensional EMG Detection in Pinnate Muscles

In pinnate muscles, such as the gastrocnemius, the fibers connect two tendon layers, called the aponeurosis, and are inclined with respect to the skin surface. As shown in Figs. 3.13 and 3.14, in a pinnate

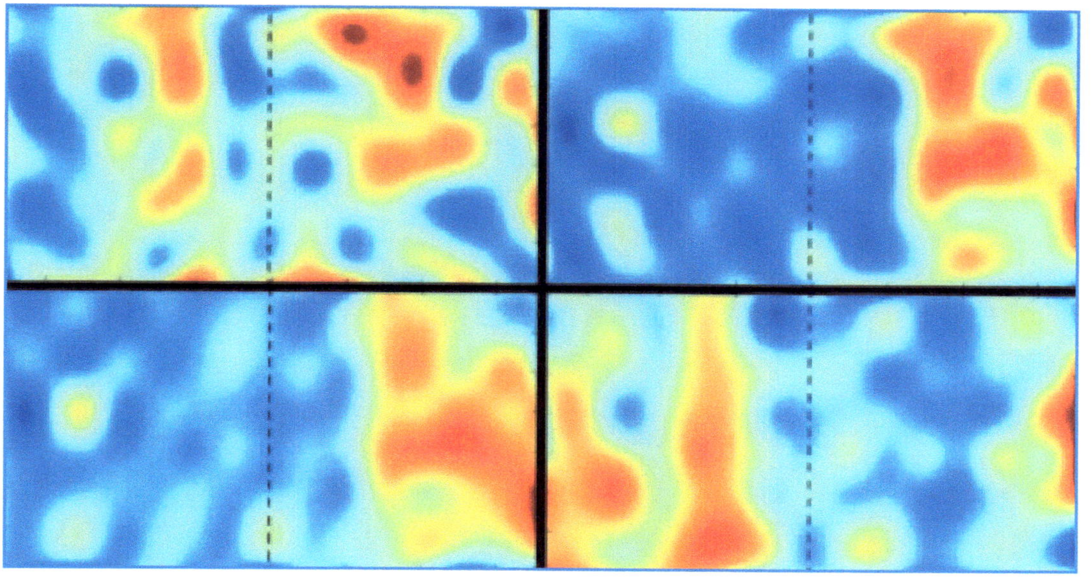

Fig. 4.7 Four sequential interpolated maps of the instantaneous LSD potentials obtained from an array of 8 rows and 16 columns placed on the gastrocnemius muscle. The *vertical dashed line* represents the boundary between the medial (*left*) and lateral (*right*) gastrocnemius. The maps are 2 ms apart, like those in Figs. 4.4 and 4.5. Due to the pinnation angle, neither the IZ nor the propagating phenomenon is visible. The potential distribution mostly reflects end-of-fiber effects (depicted also in Figs. 3.13 and 3.14) and shows where the MUAPs are extinguished at the superficial aponeurosis

muscle the monopolar or the single differential superficial potential distribution reflects mostly the end-of-fiber effect and not the propagation of MUAPs. In these muscles, larger potentials indicate a local concentration of fiber terminations belonging to the same MU, as indicated in Fig. 3.14. Therefore, the propagating potentials depicted in Figs. 4.4c and 4.5c cannot be expected on the skin above a pinnate muscle, except in particular regions, as indicated in Fig. 3.15. Figure 4.7 shows four frames, 2 ms apart, interpolated from maps obtained from an array of 8 × 16 electrodes placed over the gastrocnemius during moderate isometric contractions. The vertical dashed line indicates the separation between the gastrocnemius medialis (left) and lateralis (right). No IZ or propagation is visible and the conduction velocity cannot be estimated from these signals.

## Suggested Reading

De Nooij R, Kallenberg LA, Hermens HJ (2009) Evaluating the effect of electrode location on surface EMG amplitude of the m. erector spinae p. longissimus dorsi. J Electromyogr Kinesiol 19(4):e257-266. doi: 10.1016/j.jelekin.2008.03.013

Disselhorst-Klug C, Silny J, Rau G (1997) Improvement of spatial resolution in surface-EMG: a theoretical and experimental comparison of different spatial filters. IEEE Trans Biomed Eng 44:567-574

Jensen C, Vasseljen O, Westgaard RH (1993) The influence of electrode position on bipolar surface electromyogram recordings of the upper trapezius muscle. Eur J Appl Physiol 67:266-273

Hermens HJ, Freriks B, Disselhorst-Klug C, Rau G (2000) Development of recommendations for SEMG sensors and sensor placement procedures. J Electromyogr Kinesiol 10:361-374

Martin S, Mac Isaac D (2006) Innervation zone shift with changes in joint angle in the brachial biceps. J Electromyogr Kinesiol 16:144-148

Merletti R, Holobar A, Farina D (2008) Analysis of motor units with high-density surface electromyography. J Electromyogr Kinesiol 18:879-890

Mesin L, Merletti R, Rainoldi A (2009) Surface EMG: the issue of electrode location. J Electromyogr Kinesiol 19:719-726

Rau G, Disselhorst-Klug C (1997) Principles of high-spatial-resolution surface EMG (HSR-EMG): single motor unit detection and application in the diagnosis of neuromuscular disorders. J Electromyogr Kinesiol 7:233-239

# Features of the Single-Channel sEMG Signal

5

**Abstract**

The definitions and physiological implications of the classical amplitude (average rectified value or root mean square) and spectral features (mean or median frequency) of a single EMG channel are introduced together with the concepts of Fourier analysis and the spectrum of a signal. The spatial distribution of these quantities along an electrode array placed above the muscle is discussed. In addition, the importance of deriving these quantities from the sEMG signal collected from an area away from the innervation zone of the muscle is explained.

## 5.1 Interferential EMG Signals

A motor neuron and the muscle fibers it innervates form a motor unit (MU). Each MU is made up of dozens to hundreds of muscle fibers, and a muscle, in turn, is made up of dozens to hundreds of MUs. Figure 5.1a schematically shows two MUs of a few fibers each. As indicated in the previous chapters, each muscle fiber contributes to the signal detected by surface electrodes with a single action potential (AP), as shown in Fig. 5.1b. The superficial APs generated by fibers belonging to the same MU add up to form the motor unit action potential (MUAP), also indicated in Fig. 5.1b. Examples of many multichannel MUAPs are provided in Figs. 3.8 and 3.9.

Each active MU discharges at a rate of 6–8 to 30–40 times per second, depending on its central drive, generating a MUAP train. Multiple MUAP trains together form an interferential EMG signal, depicted in Fig. 5.1c. This signal has features that depend on anatomical and physiological parameters (the number of active MUs and the discharge rate of each one, the thickness of the subcutaneous tissue, the orientation of the MUs) as well as on detection parameters (location, area, and spacing of the electrodes). Additional information on the role of these factors is provided in the literature (Farina et al., 2002a).

## 5.2 Amplitude Features of EMG Signals: Single-Channel

Consider the 1D signal segment depicted in Fig. 4.1a. Its "instantaneous amplitude" is different for any time sample. Can we define an "average amplitude" that allows comparison among different signals and provides an indication of which signal is larger and which is smaller? The concept of averaging is associated with a time window; that is, we speak of an average over a specified time interval, referred to as a signal "epoch."

The average amplitude of any EMG signal computed over epochs longer than about 0.1 s is zero since the signal is the sum of zero-mean MUAPs and has equal likelihoods of being positive or negative. To avoid this problem, the "absolute value" of the signal is considered, defined as the instantaneous value, which is always taken to be positive even when it is negative. This new signal is also called "rectified" because it has a single polarity, since the negative swings are consid-

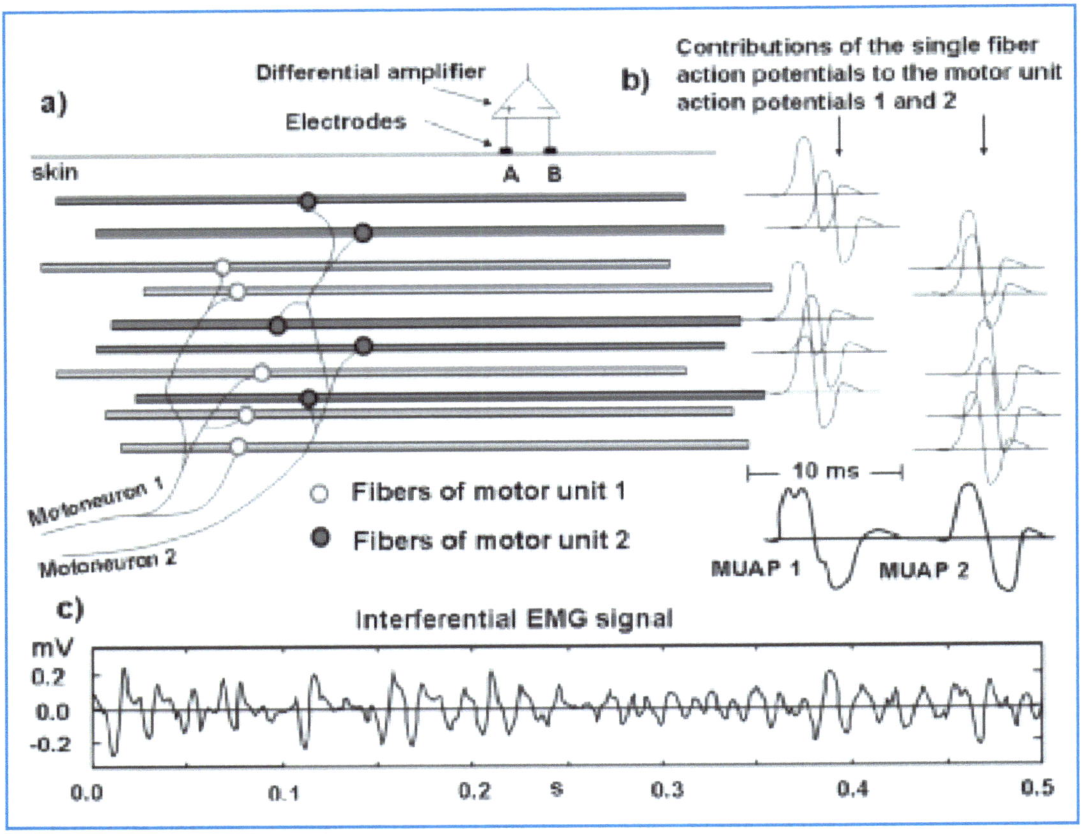


**Fig. 5.1** **a** Example of two motor units in a fusiform muscle with fibers parallel to the skin. **b** The APs of the individual fibers as differentially detected by electrodes A and B and their sum generating the respective motor unit action potentials (MUAPs). **c** Interferential EMG signal differentially detected by electrodes A and B when hundreds of MUAPs contribute to the signal. The mean value of the APs is zero, as is the mean value of the interferential signal

ered to be positive. The average of the rectified EMG signal is called the average rectified value (ARV). It is defined over an epoch of specified duration and is a "variable" (not a parameter) of the EMG signal that changes from epoch to epoch. This value is also called the mean rectified value (MRV) or mean absolute value (MAV). For a multichannel signal, the ARV is defined for each channel, for the same epoch duration. Epoch durations range from 0.125 s to 1–2 s depending on whether the signal properties are changing slowly or quickly. Figure 5.2a shows an epoch of 150 ms of one channel of an interferential EMG signal, and Fig. 5.2b the rectified value (solid line) and its average value (dashed line).

An alternative amplitude feature is the root mean squared value (RMS), a short expression for the "square root of the mean squared value." In this case, depicted in Fig. 5.3, the instantaneous signal is squared (solid line in Fig. 5.3b), yielding a signal that is never negative. The average of this signal is then the mean square value (MSV) and its square root is the RMS, indicated by a dashed line in Fig. 5.3b.

Both the ARV and RMS fluctuate from epoch to epoch because signals generated in different epochs are affected by random factors, but they show no trend if the signal is "stationary". By contrast, the presence of a trend in time indicates that some physiological quantity is progressively changing in time and affecting the superficial signal's amplitude. Progressive changes in a muscle

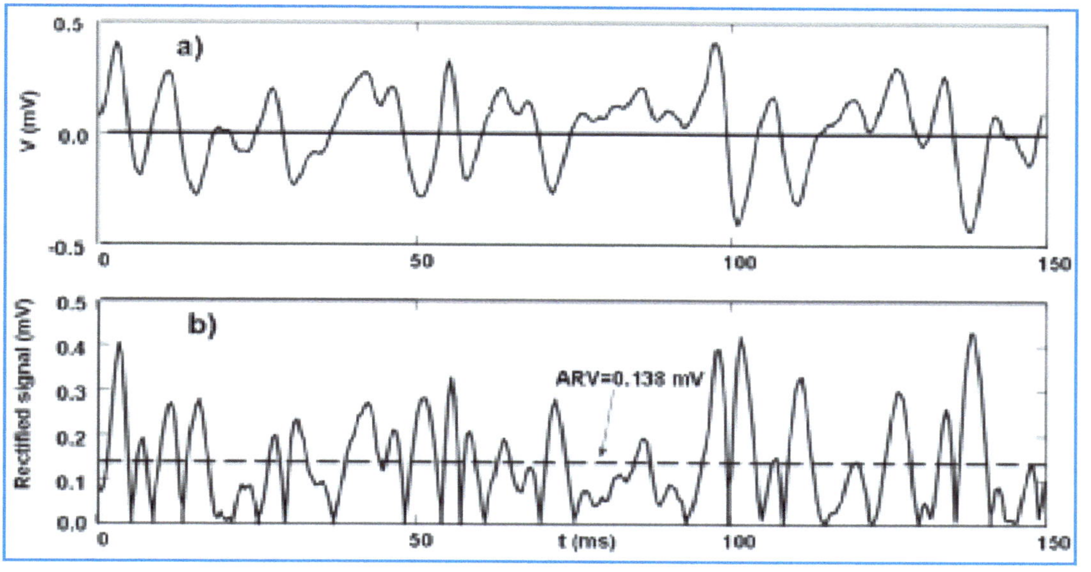


**Fig. 5.2** **a** Example of an interferential EMG signal detected by one electrode pair during an epoch of 150 ms. **b** The signal depicted in **a** is "rectified" (*solid line*) and its average is computed. The average rectified value (*ARV*) is indicated by the *dashed line* and may differ from epoch to epoch. If the ARV shows a trend from epoch to epoch the signal is said to be non-stationary

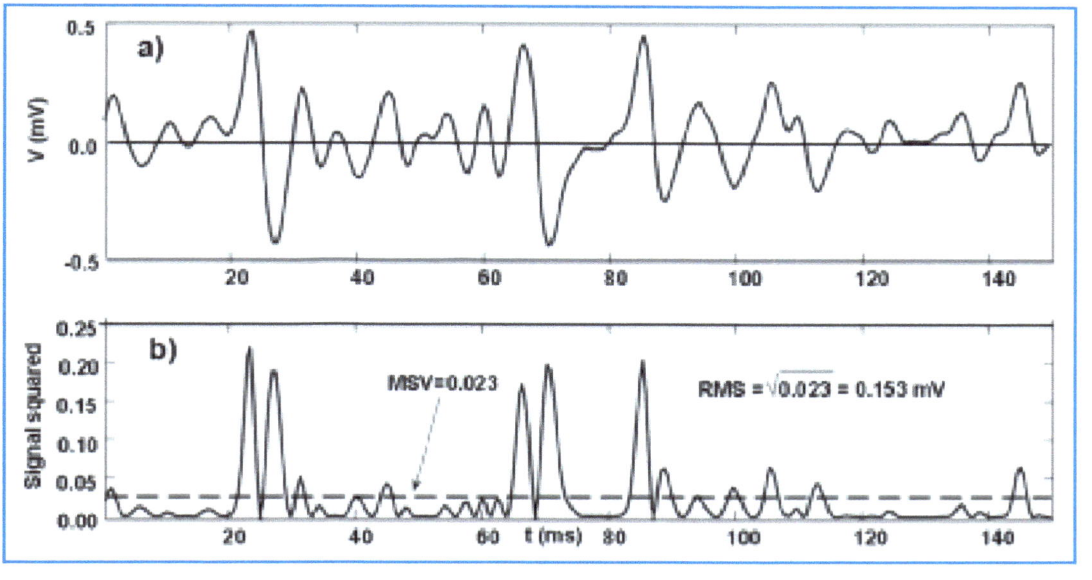


**Fig. 5.3** **a** Example of an interferential EMG signal detected by one electrode pair during an epoch of 150 ms. **b** The signal depicted in **a** is "squared" (*solid line*) and its average is computed. The mean squared value (*MSV*) is indicated by the *dashed line* and its square root is the root mean square (*RMS*), the value of which may differ from epoch to epoch. If the RMS shows a trend from epoch to epoch the signal is said to be non-stationary

fiber's conduction velocity or the spatial width of a single fiber potential, or changes in the discharge rate or the recruitment or derecruitment of MUs are all factors that produce trends.

Both the ARV and the RMS are strongly affected by the location of the electrodes with respect to the innervation zone(s) and tendon endings in fusiform muscles with fibers parallel to the skin. In pinnate muscles, changes in the ARV and RMS reflect changes of signal amplitude due to the end-of-fiber effect.

The ARV and RMS carry very similar information and are often used interchangeably. A different rate of change (that is, a change in the ratio) of these two variables in time, however, indicates a change in the shape of the probability density function of the signal and a particular type of nonstationarity. If the change in the signal properties (trends) is slow, and therefore negligible within each epoch, the signal is "quasi-stationary". Nonstationary signals and their properties are not addressed in this book.

## 5.3 Basic Concepts of Analysis in the Frequency Domain

Sinusoids or sine waves in space and time were discussed in Chapter 2 and are analyzed in greater detail in this section. A sinusoid is a mathematical function, described in Fig. 5.4a, whose general equation is $y = A \sin \alpha$ , where $\alpha$ is an angle expressed in radians. This function is generated by a rotating segment of length A whose angle with the x axis is $\alpha$ and where $\sin \alpha$ is B/A. As the segment rotates around the origin at a constant angu-

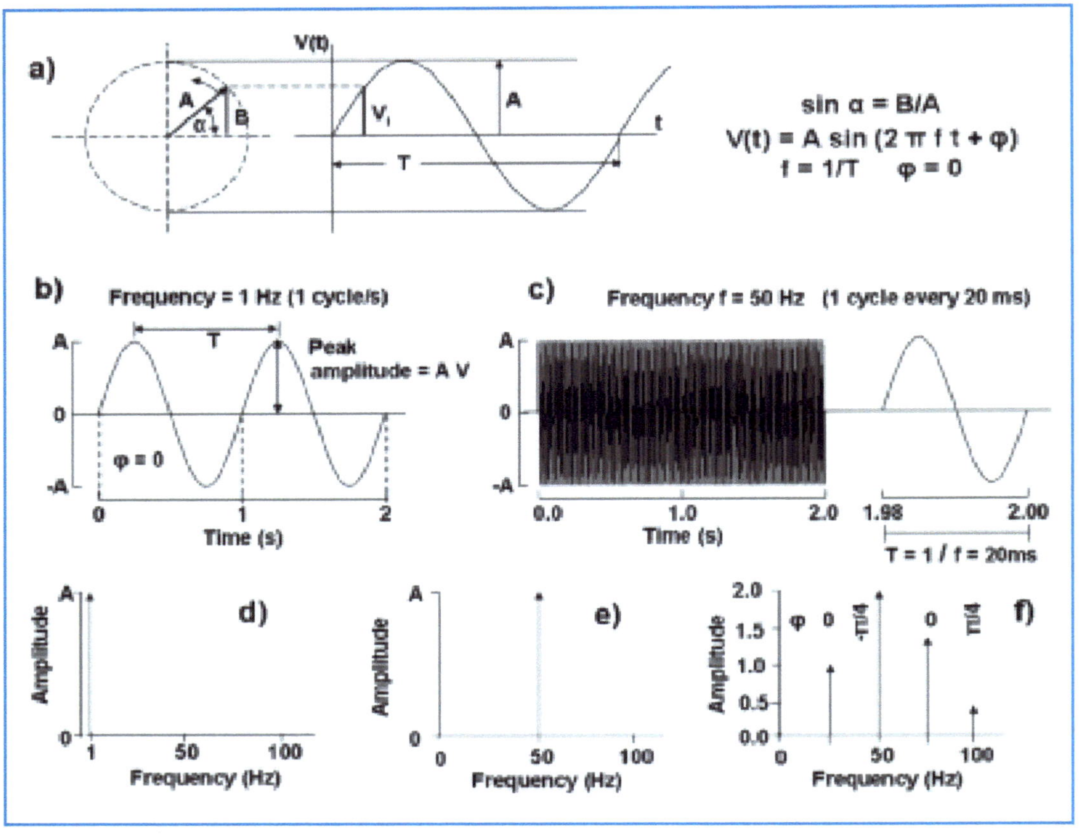


**Fig. 5.4** a Generation of a sinusoidal function given by the length of segment B vs. time as vector A rotates counter-clockwise with a velocity of $2\pi f$ radians/s starting from angle $\phi$ ($\phi = 0$ in this case). b, c Two sinusoids, having a frequency of 1 Hz and 50 Hz, respectively, and represented in the time domain. d, e Representation of the two frequencies in the frequency domain (amplitude spectrum). f Amplitude and phase spectrum of a signal composed of four sinusoids having amplitudes of 1, 2, 1.5, and 0.5 V and frequencies of 25, 50, 75, and 100 Hz, respectively

lar velocity, the length of segment B describes a curve in time that swings between +A and –A, as depicted in Fig. 5.4a, and whose equation is $y = A \sin(2\pi ft + \phi)$, where $(2\pi ft + \phi) = \alpha$, A is the amplitude or peak value, f is the frequency, and $\phi$ the phase of the function (i.e., the initial angle of the rotating segment at $t = 0$).

When y is a signal in time (i.e., a voltage), the equation becomes $V(t) = A \sin(2\pi ft + \phi)$, where V(t) is the instantaneous value $V_i$ that is changing in time. The frequency is the number of cycles per second and the duration of a cycle is T, so that $f = 1/T$ or $T = 1/f$. The rotating velocity in radians/s is $2\pi f$ (one cycle is $2\pi$ radians). T is measured in seconds (s) and f in cycles per second, or Hertz (Hz); $\phi$ is the starting angle (at t =0) and is measured in radians. Figure 5.4b, c shows a sinusoid having a frequency of 1 Hz (T = 1s) and another with a frequency of 50 Hz (T=0.020 s = 20 ms), both having a peak value A.

An alternative way to represent sinusoids is depicted in Fig 5.4a, d, where the horizontal axis shows the frequency and the vertical axis the amplitude of the wave. The two sinusoids of Fig. 5.4b, c are then represented by the two lines indicated in Fig. 5.4d, e.

Figure 5.4f describes a signal that is made up of four sinusoids having, respectively, peak values of 1.0, 2.0, 1.5, and 0.5 V frequencies of 25, 50, 75, and 100 Hz, and phases $\phi$ of 0, $-\pi/4$, 0, and $+\pi/4$ radians (corresponding to 0, -90, 0, and +90°). What would a signal formed by the sum of these four sinusoids look like? Figure 5.5a shows these four sinusoids and their sum. We can say that the signal at the bottom is the sum of the four sinusoids or that it can be "decomposed" into the four sinusoids that comprise it. We can also observe that the sum signal is no longer a sinusoid but is periodic, with a period equal to that of the first sinusoid (the one with the lowest frequency).

The "power" of a signal is the energy produced per unit time when this signal is applied to a unitary resistor; it is equal to the MSV of the signal, which is the square of the RMS value (see Fig. 5.3). For a sinusoid, the MSV is the square of the peak value divided by 2. Figure 5.5b shows the power contributed to the signal by each of its four sinusoidal components (harmonics). This diagram is called the "power spectrum" of the signal and it is obtained by plotting, as vertical bars or arrows, the power contributed to the signal by each of the harmonics, the frequencies of which are indicated on the horizontal axis.

A signal is said to be described in the time domain when it is represented as in Fig. 5.2a, 5.3a, 5.4b, or 5.5a. A signal is said to be described in the frequency domain when it is represented as in Fig. 5.4f (amplitude and phase spectrum) or as in Fig. 5.5b (power spectrum), when we describe it in terms of the sum of sinusoids.

Indeed, the concepts introduced above can be generalized. Any periodic signal can be described as the sum of sinusoids, called harmonics. The first harmonic (also called the fundamental harmonic) has the same frequency as the original periodic signal while the other harmonics have frequencies that are multiples of the fundamental. The sinusoids depicted in Fig. 5.5 are the harmonics of the signal shown at the bottom of Fig. 5.5a. Breaking down a periodic signal into its harmonics is called a "Fourier analysis." Figure 5.4f shows a Fourier analysis (amplitude spectrum) of the signal depicted at the bottom of Fig. 5.5a. Figure 5.5b shows the power spectrum of the same signal.

The Fourier analysis applies also to non-periodic signals, with the implicit assumption that the available signal epoch (such as that depicted in Fig. 5.2a or 5.3a) repeats periodically, so that the "new" signal becomes "periodic." This fact is obviously not true in the case of bioelectric signals, but has no consequences on the physiological interpretation of the signal's spectrum. A new spectrum is computed for every signal epoch and it changes from epoch to epoch. It is important to underline that if a signal epoch has duration T, the first harmonic will have a frequency 1/T , the second harmonic a frequency of 2/T, the third a frequency 3/T, and so on. The harmonics are therefore separated by 1/T Hz, so that an EMG signal epoch of 0.5s will produce a spectrum whose harmonics are separated by 2 Hz while an EMG signal epoch of 0.1s will produce a spectrum whose harmonics are separated by 10 Hz. It is therefore clear that very short epochs generate a poorly defined spectrum with few harmonics spaced very far apart (low-frequency resolution) whereas a

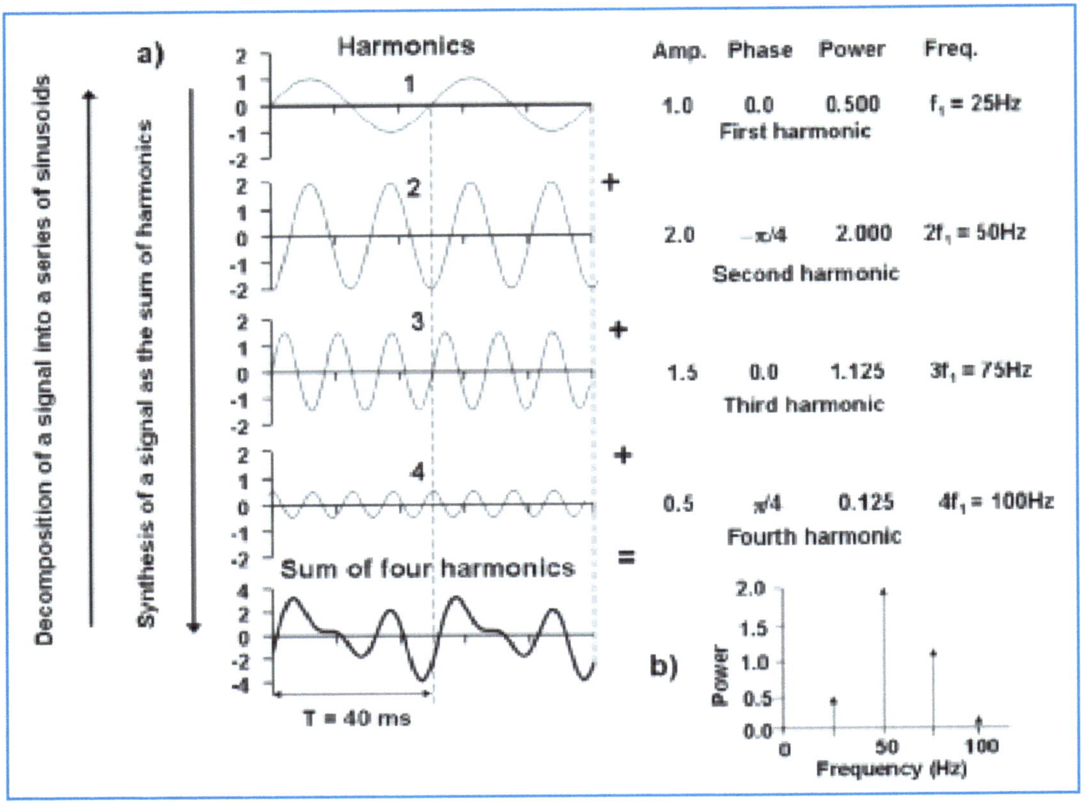


**Fig. 5.5** The signal described in the frequency domain (amplitude and phase spectra) in Fig. 5.4f is depicted here in the time domain. **a** The four sinusoidal components (harmonics of the signal) are depicted together with their sum. **b** The power spectrum, describing the power contribution of each harmonic to the total power, is shown. The power of each harmonic is the mean square value of the corresponding sinusoid, which is the square of the amplitude (peak value) divided by 2

long epoch (e.g., 2 s) generates a well-defined spectrum with many harmonics separated by 0.5 Hz (high-frequency resolution).

It is also intuitive that a complex signal, such as an EMG epoch of 0.25–1.0 s duration, will have many harmonics because many sinusoids will be required to reconstruct this irregular signal. Note that the harmonics obtained through Fourier analysis have no physiological counterpart or meaning. No sinusoidal signals are produced by muscles or other organs; rather, the harmonics, and the spectrum of a signal that they form, are simply a mathematical tool. The usefulness of this tool is described in the next section.

The spectrum of an audio signal (e.g., a music segment) is often depicted by audio reproduction devices, in which the spectrum is presented as a histogram. Each "bin" of the histogram includes a few harmonics and the frequency range covers the bandwidth of the audio signals (20–5000 Hz or 20–10000 Hz). The power spectrum of a music epoch in which drums, horns, or other low-pitch instruments are dominant is shown in Fig. 5.6a, and the power spectrum of a music epoch in which violins, flutes, or other high-pitch instruments are dominant in Fig. 5.6b. Indeed, the musical notes are a form of spectral description of a musical sound (different from the Fourier description). The "notes" contained in the sEMG signal are of very low pitch, ranging from 20 to about 400 Hz; if the signal is fed to an amplifier and a loudspeaker, the sound produced is a low rumble, very different from that produced by the signal detected with intramuscular needles, which has a much higher pitch and in which the "clicks" of MU discharges can be heard.

## 5.4 The Concept of the Power Spectrum and the Spectral Features of the Surface Single-Channel EMG Signal

Each of the signals depicted in Figs. 3.9, 3.10, 5.1c, 5.2a, and 5.3a represents one epoch of a sEMG recording. Fourier analysis of many epochs of sEMG recordings shows that 95–99% of the power of the EMG signal is contributed by harmonics in the frequency range of 10–20 Hz to 350–400 Hz. The power spectrum (often simply referred to as the "spectrum") of the sEMG has the typical shape indicated in Figs. 5.6c and 5.8c. Since the signal is random and no two signal epochs are identical, the estimated spectrum has random fluctuations from epoch to epoch.

During sustained or intermittent fatiguing contractions, the spectrum shows a trend in time and the EMG is therefore non-stationary. The quantification of these trends is important in order to evaluate myoelectric manifestations of muscle fatigue and requires the definition of "features," which are variables whose change in time provides a simple quantitative description of the progressive spectral changes. Many such features have been defined and discussed in the literature (e.g., with respect to the number of zero crossings or the number of "turns" in the epoch considered) but the most widely used features are the mean frequency (MNF) and the median frequency (MDF) (De Luca, 1984). The MNF is also called the mean spectral frequency (MSF), centroid frequency, or "first moment" frequency. The MDF is sometimes called the 50$^{th}$ percentile frequency. MNF and MDF are defined as follows and are depicted in Fig. 5.6c, where the vertical lines represent the harmonics that define the spectrum.

The MNF, or centroid frequency, is the center of gravity line of the spectrum. Let us imagine that the spectrum depicted in Fig. 5.6c is cut out of a piece of cardboard and balanced on a blade parallel to the power axis. The blade location that balances the spectrum is called the "centroid line," or the mean frequency of the spectrum. It must be underlined that the name may be misleading. Indeed, the mean frequency is not the mean of any frequencies: it is the frequency corresponding to the centroid, or center of gravity, of the spectrum.

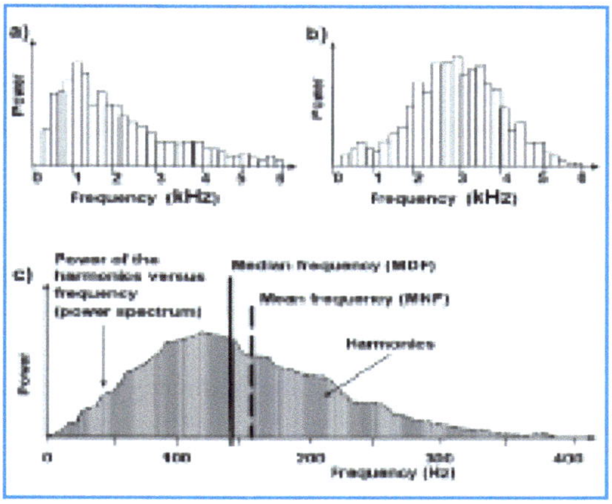


**Fig. 5.6** Power spectrum, presented in the form of a histogram, of a piece of music played on low-pitch instruments (**a**) or high-pitch instruments (**b**). **c** Power spectrum of an epoch of the sEMG monopolar signal. The *vertical hatching* represents the harmonics. At an epoch length of 2 s, the harmonics would be 0.5 Hz apart and there would be 800 harmonics in the 0–400 Hz frequency range. At an epoch length of 0.5 s, the harmonics would be 2 Hz apart and there would be 200 harmonics in the 0–400 Hz frequency range. Half of the power carried by the harmonics (whatever their number) is below the MDF and the other half above it. The MNF is the line corresponding to the center of gravity (or centroid) of the spectrum

The MDF is the frequency at which half of the power of the signal is below it (harmonics lower than the MDF) and half is above it (harmonics higher than the MDF). In other words, the harmonics below the MDF account for half the signal power and those above it for the other half. Note that this does not mean that half of the harmonics are below the MDF and half are above it. The MNF and MDF coincide in the case of a spectrum symmetric with respect to its midline. The MNF is greater than the MDF if the spectrum is skewed to the right. This is usually the case in sEMG (see Fig. 5.6c).

The spectral variables (MNF and MDF) are related to a number of physiological variables, which include the conduction velocity of the APs along the fibers (Farina et al., 2002a).

Consider the concepts describing a source moving below two sensors, as explained in Sect. 2.4.

The example given in Fig. 2.6 can be applied to each of the harmonics of the EMG signal. If the sinusoid in space described in Fig. 2.6 moves more slowly under the electrodes, the sinusoid in time detected by each of the two electrodes will last longer in time; that is, its period T increases and its frequency decreases (in Sect. 2.4, it is shown that $f = 1/T = v/\lambda$, where $\lambda$ is the wavelength of the sinusoid in space). Consequently, a 10% decrement of the conduction velocity of an AP will imply a 10% decrement of the frequency of each of the harmonics of the spectrum of that potential, and therefore of the MNF and MDF. In conclusion, either spectral variable (MNF or MDF) can provide information on the changes of the conduction velocity of an AP. A decrement of this velocity would therefore result in an equivalent percent change in the MNF or MDF that is easier to estimate and requires a single EMG channel, while the estimation of conduction velocity requires multiple channels (see Figs. 3.7, 3.8). Unfortunately, in general, things are much more complicated, even for muscles with fibers parallel to the skin, and the operator's awareness of these complications is important.

For example, consider again the case described in Sect. 2.4 and Fig. 2.6. A sine wave, propagating in space with velocity v and having wavelength $\lambda = d$, where d is the interelectrode distance (IED) of a differential detection system, would provide no output. Such a sine wave in space would have a corresponding sine wave in time (appearing at the output of the differential system) of frequency $f = v/\lambda$. Therefore, because of the differential detection (that is, because of the differential spatial filter), the spectrum of the differential signal would have a "dip" down to zero at this frequency. Considering a typical conduction velocity of 4 m/s and an IED of d = 10 mm, the dip would appear at 4/0.01 = 400 Hz, that is, at the edge of the spectrum, and would not greatly influence it. However, for the more frequently used IED of 20 mm, the dip would be at 200 Hz and the shape of the spectrum would be greatly modified. Again, things are more complicated than this, since different MUs have fibers with somewhat different conduction velocities. Each MU would produce a dip at a spectral frequency somewhat different from the others, and the resulting multiple dips would smooth out and often would not be visible in the spectrum of a differential signal.

From these considerations, it can be concluded that the spectrum of a longitudinal single differential (LSD) EMG signal strongly depends on the IED and on the electrode's location above a muscle. Therefore, amplitude and spectral variables are also affected such that a comparison between signal features measured with different electrode locations or IEDs is not only meaningless but may be highly misleading.

A practical example is reported in Fig. 5.7 for the trapezius muscle. This example clearly shows how widely different the values of ARV and MNF can be as we move along a muscle in the fiber direction with one pair of electrodes and how critical the location of the electrodes and their distance can be. At locations where the signal is small, the noise generated by the electrode-skin junctions and by the amplifier becomes relevant. Since the spectrum of the noise is wider than that of the sEMG signal, the total spectrum of the sEMG plus noise is wider than that of the sEMG alone and the MNF and MDF values are higher, as shown in Fig. 5.7c. Indeed, the only "good" electrode location in the case shown in this figure is at about 45% of the C7–acromion distance, starting from the acromion. Even in this location, the variation of the IED from 5 mm to 40 mm increases the ARV by a factor of five and decreases the MNF by more than 20%. A more detailed description and analysis of these large changes is provided in the literature (Farina, 2002; Beck et al., 2007, 2008, 2009; Hermens and Freriks, 1997).

During a muscle contraction of sustained constant force, the muscle fiber AP conduction velocity changes, as do the MU firing frequencies and the degree of their synchronization. Some MUs may drop out and new ones may be recruited. All these changes cause variations in the amplitude and spectral features of the EMG signal and in its spectral shape. Together they provide the "myoelectric manifestations of muscle fatigue" that precede the "mechanical manifestations of muscle fatigue," that is, the inability to further sustain the required force level.

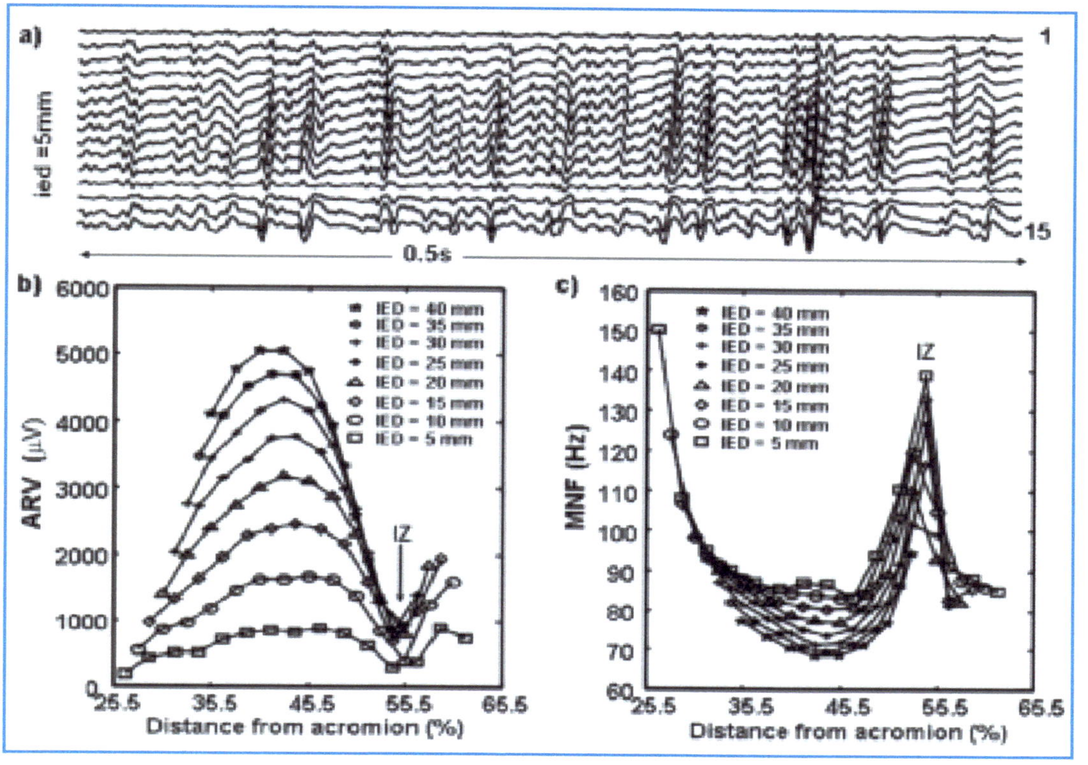


Fig. 5.7 **a** The sEMG signals detected from the upper trapezius muscle during isometric abduction of the arms at 90° with a bilateral hand load of 1 kg. The signals are recorded by a linear array of 16 electrodes in LSD mode, with an interelectrode distance (IED) of 5 mm. A single innervation zone (IZ) can be clearly detected under channel 12–13. **b, c** Values of ARV and MNF as functions of electrode location and the IED for the signals shown in **a** and computed on a 0.5 s epoch. Signals corresponding to different IEDs are obtained by adding the single differential signals between the first and last electrodes of interest. The distance from the acromion is indicated as a percentage of the acromion–C7 length. The IZ is located in the region between 50% and 60% of the distance acromion–C7, starting from the acromion. The "good" region for placing a pair of electrodes is between 40% and 50% of the distance acromion–C7, starting from the acromion (reprinted from Farina et al.,2002b)

Two interferential single differential (SD) EMG signal epochs of 0.5 s each, detected at the beginning and end of a long, sustained, constant-force isometric contraction of the biceps brachii (IED = 20 mm), are depicted in Fig. 5.8a, b. Their different "frequency contents" are readily visible (the second signal is "slower" than the first) and are reflected by the different spectra. In most cases, the main cause of this modification is a reduction of the AP conduction velocity, which increases the time duration of their superficial contributions to the sEMG. In this case, the spectrum would be "scaled" or "compressed" in time to the left (as a retracting rubber band) and "scaled" in amplitude because of the increased area under the MUAPs. In Fig. 5.8c, the spectrum of signal 2 is indeed an approximate scaled version of the spectrum of signal 1. The percentage decrement in the MNF or MDF would equal the percent decrement of the conduction velocity and the changes of the spectral variables would reflect those of the conduction velocity. In general, they would reflect not only the changes of conduction velocity but also those of other variables (active MU pool, AP shapes, etc.). A careful observer may note and interpret the spectral "dip" at about 180 Hz and associate it with the previous considerations. Such dips are difficult to observe and quite often are not evident at all. The discussion of the effects of the anatomic, physiologic, and geometric parameters on indices of my-

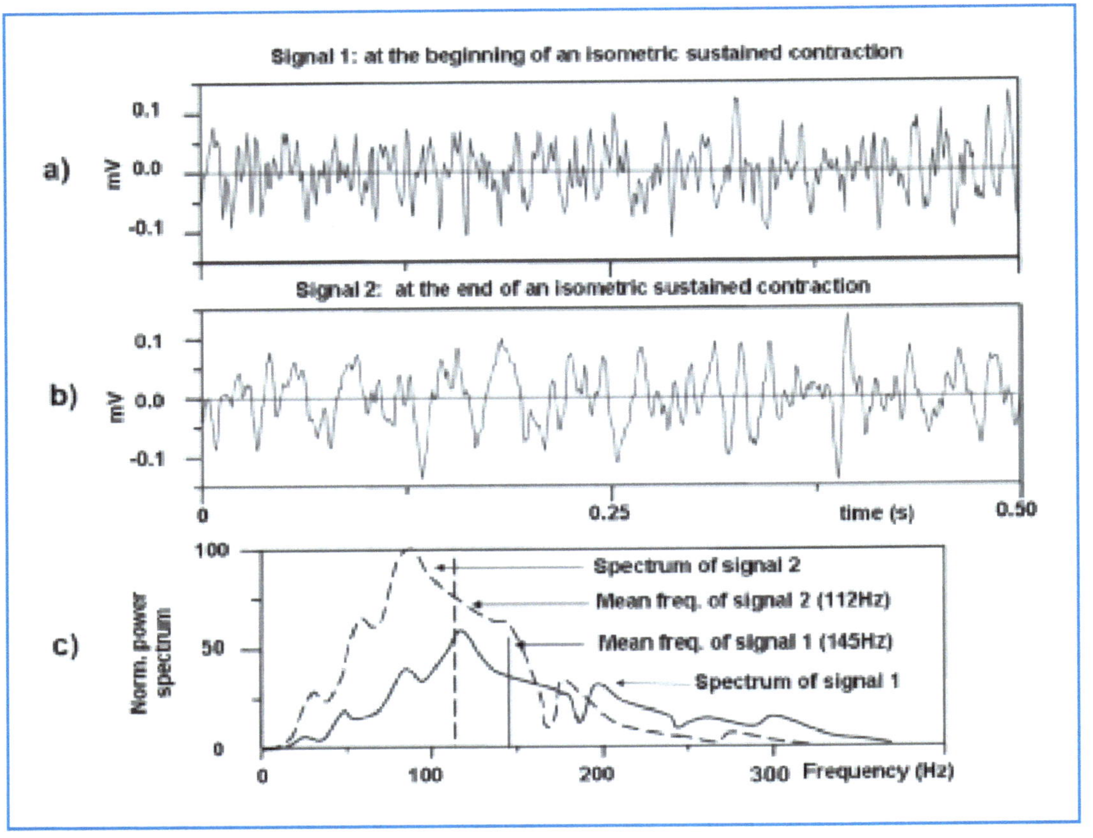


**Fig. 5.8** Examples of two epochs of interferential LSD EMG signals recorded at the beginning and at the end of a fatiguing, isometric, constant-force muscle contraction of the biceps brachii. **a** Initial epoch, **b** final epoch, **c** normalized spectra (the amplitude of the largest harmonic is defined as 100 and the others are shown as percentages thereof) obtained from the two signal epochs. For clarity, the harmonics are not represented. The evident "spectral compression" is one of the most important "myoelectric manifestations of muscle fatigue"

oelectric manifestations of muscle fatigue exceeds the objectives of this book, but is reported in the literature (Farina et al., 2002a, b; Karlsson et al., 2009; De Luca, 1984; Kupa et al.,1995; Mannion et al., 1998; Kallenberg et al., 2007; Rainoldi et al., 2008; Farina et al., 2003).

Figure 5.9 depicts the progression of the spectral changes manifested by a LSD EMG channel during a contraction sustained to endurance (90 s). For clarity, only four spectra, 30s apart, are depicted, with each one calculated over the indicated signal epoch. The centroid lines defining the MNF values are shown and the MNF pattern of variation in time is outlined. It is interesting to note that the MNF starts to change from the very beginning of the contraction while the inability to sustain force (mechanical manifestation of muscle fatigue) occurs at the endurance time (90 s). It should now be obvious that the features of the signals depicted in Figs. 5.8 and 5.9 would have been different if another electrode location or IED had been chosen.

The concepts and examples illustrated in this section and in Figs. 5.6, 5.8, and 5.9 concern a single sEMG signal (one channel). Figure 5.7 shows the much greater wealth of information provided by a linear electrode array vs. a single pair of electrodes (concerning the estimation of average AP conduction velocity, IZ location, etc.). It should now be easy to extrapolate these concepts to a 2D grid of electrodes. These issues are addressed in Chapter 6.

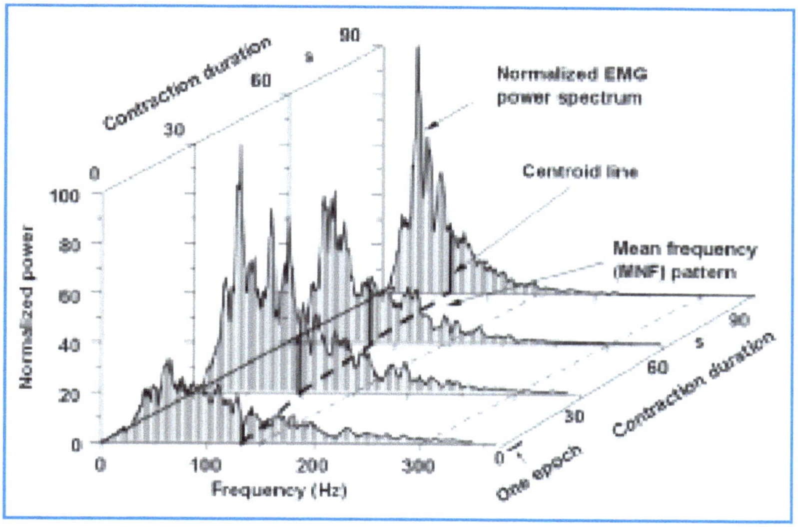


**Fig. 5.9** Progressive spectral compression of a LSD EMG signal detected from a biceps brachii during a fatiguing isometric contraction sustained for 90 s. The *hatching* represents the harmonics. The force produced by the muscle is constant until the endurance point (90 s) but the EMG signal spectrum changes considerably already at the beginning of the contraction and its mean frequency (MNF) decreases from 130 to 60 Hz

## Suggested Reading


Beck TW, Housh TJ, Mielke M et al (2007) The influence of electrode placement over the innervation zone on electromyographic amplitude and mean power frequency versus isokinetic torque relationships. J Neurosci Meth 162:72-83

Beck TW, Housh TJ, Cramer, JT, Weir JP (2008) The effects of electrode placement and innervation zone location on the electromyographic amplitude and mean power frequency versus isometric torque relationships for the vastus lateralis muscle. J Electromyogr Kinesiol 18:317-328

Beck TW, Housh TJ, Cramer JT et al (2009) Electrode placement over the innervation zone affects the low, not the high-frequency portion of the EMG frequency spectrum. J Electromyogr Kinesiol 19:660-666

De Luca CJ (1984) Myoelectrical manifestations of localized muscular fatigue in humans. Crit Rev Biomed Eng 11:251-279

Farina D, Cescon C, Merletti R (2002a) Influence of anatomical, physical, and detection-system parameters on surface EMG. Biol Cybern. 86:445-56

Farina D, Madeline P, Graven-Nielsen T et al (2002b) Standardising surface electromyogram recordings for assessment of activity and fatigue in the human upper trapezius muscle. Eur J Appl Physiol 86:469-478

Farina D, Kallenberg LA, Merletti R, Hermens HJ (2003) Effect of side dominance on myoelectric manifestations of muscle fatigue in the human upper trapezius muscle. Eur J Appl Physiol 90:480-488

Hermens HJ, Freriks B (1997) SENIAM 5: The State of the Art on Sensors and Sensor Placement Procedures for Surface ElectroMyoGraphy: A proposal for sensor placement procedures. Roessingh Research and Development, Enschede, NL

Kallenberg LA, Schulte E, Disselhorst-Klug C, Hermens HJ (2007) Myoelectric manifestations of fatigue at low contraction levels in subjects with and without chronic pain. J Electromyogr Kinesiol 17:264-274

Karlsson S, Roeleveld K, Gronlund C et al (2009) Signal processing of the surface electromyogram to gain insight into neuromuscular physiology. Philos Transact A Math Phys Eng Sci 367:337-356

Kupa EJ, Roy SH, Kandarian SC, De Luca CJ (1995) Effects of muscle fiber type and size on EMG median frequency and conduction velocity. J Appl Physiol 79:23-32

Mannion AF, Dumas GA, Stevenson JM, Cooper RG (1998) The influence of muscle fiber size and type distribution on electromyographic measures of back muscle fatigability. Spine 23:576-584

Rainoldi A, Falla D, Mellor R et al (2008) Myoelectric manifestations of fatigue in vastus lateralis, medialis obliquus and medialis longus muscles. J Electromyogr Kinesiol 18:1032-1037

# 6 Features of the Two-Dimensional sEMG Signal: EMG Feature Imaging

**Abstract**

The concept of the time-varying spatial distribution of the instantaneous EMG potential on the skin above a muscle is extended to the maps of EMG features. Applications to the interpretation of averaged amplitude maps and of maps of spectral variables are outlined, with a few examples. The utility of these maps in the study of muscles and in the identification of electrode locations is discussed. Common mistakes and pitfalls in electrode placement are pointed out.

## 6.1 Amplitude Variables and Their Spatial Distribution

A grid of sensors can be described as a 2D array of potential detectors that provides an instantaneous image for every time sample, either as a set of pixels or as an interpolated smoothed picture. Applications to the sEMG signal are illustrated in Figs. 4.2–4.5. This concept of a 2D representation of the instantaneous EMG amplitude map can be extended to the values of sEMG features calculated for every signal epoch. Accordingly, instead of having an image of sEMG intensity for every sample, we have an image of the ARV or RMS or MNF or MDF (see Chapter 5) spatial distribution for every epoch. A signal epoch now provides a "sample," or a map or frame, of the sEMG feature of interest. However, this sample is not "instantaneous" but "integrated" over the epoch duration and associated with each epoch.

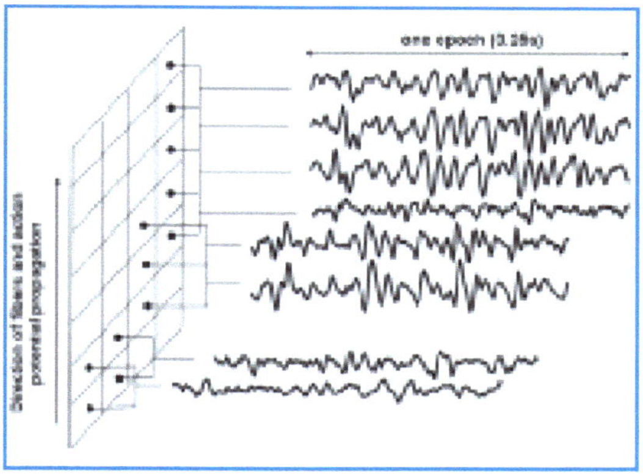

Fig. 6.1 Two dimensional electrode array and corresponding image pixels (see also Fig. 4.2b). Longitudinal (along the direction of the fibers) single differential EMG channels are shown for an epoch duration of 0.25 s. EMG features can be computed for each epoch and for each channel and their values can be attributed to the center point of each pixel. Interpolation in space (see Fig. 4.2c) provides images such as those reported in Figs. 6.2–6.8

An example is provided in Fig. 6.1. The skin surface is described by a grid of pixels, one for each electrode, providing a set of monopolar signals. The longitudinal single differential (LSD) sEMG signals are computed by taking the difference between each monopolar signal and its neighbor, along the fiber direction (columns). Let us consider an epoch (e.g., 0.25 s) of each of these LSD sEMG signals, as indicated in Fig. 6.1, and compute the amplitude and spectral features (EMG variables) of each channel for the given epoch. Each channel will then be associated with ARV, RMS, MNF, and MDF values, generating a map of values for each of these variables. A new map is thus created

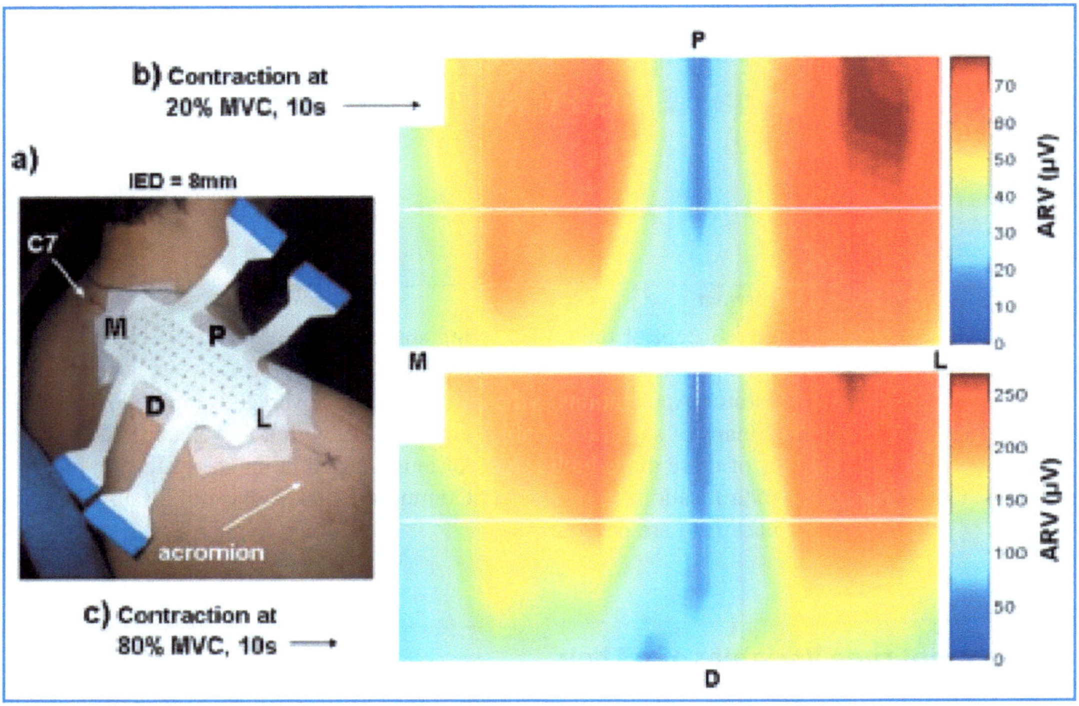


**Fig. 6.2** **a** Example of a two dimensional (2D) electrode array applied above the mid-upper trapezius during isometric constant-force contractions. *M*, medial; *L*, lateral; *P*, proximal; *D*, distal. **b, c** Interpolated maps of the ARVs of the LSD EMG computed on a 10-s epoch during 20% MVC and an 80% MVC contractions. *MVC* Maximal voluntary contraction. Note the different color scales in **b** and **c**. IED = 8 mm in both directions. *White line,* C7–acromion line

for every new epoch and displays the sEMG variables corresponding to that epoch.

The sequence of the maps will form a movie, with frames separated by the epoch duration. The same can be done for variables obtained from monopolar signals, double differential signals, or signals obtained using other spatial filters. Such map(s) could then be interpolated to generate a better picture, as in Fig. 6.2. The advantages and disadvantages of these other maps with respect to the most widely used maps obtained from single differential (SD) channels, as well as their applications, have been addressed in the literature (Farina et al., 2002; Hedayatpour et al., 2008; Tucker et al., 2009); their discussion is beyond the scope of this book.

Figure 6.2a shows a 2D electrode array (5 columns × 13 rows, IED = 8 mm) placed over a portion of the trapezius muscle with the "columns" aligned with the C7–acromion direction, which is the approximate direction of the fibers. The midpoint of the array and the midpoint of the C7–acromion line coincide. After the maximal voluntary contraction (MVC) force was measured, two contractions of 10 s duration were performed, respectively, at 20% MVC and 80% MVC. The two LSD-interpolated sEMG maps thus obtained are shown in Fig. 6.2. We can see that this subject has a well defined single innervation zone (IZ) in the middle of the array (blue area) and that the sEMG ARV is higher in the lateral than in the medial portion of the array, and in the proximal than in the distal portion of the array. Such considerations apply both at low and at high contraction levels. The peak ARV during the 10 s contraction increases from about 80 µV to about 260 µV and remains in the same location.

The raw signals (such as those depicted in Fig. 6.1) provide more detailed information (including information about individual motor units (MUs), the presence of interference or noise, etc., which

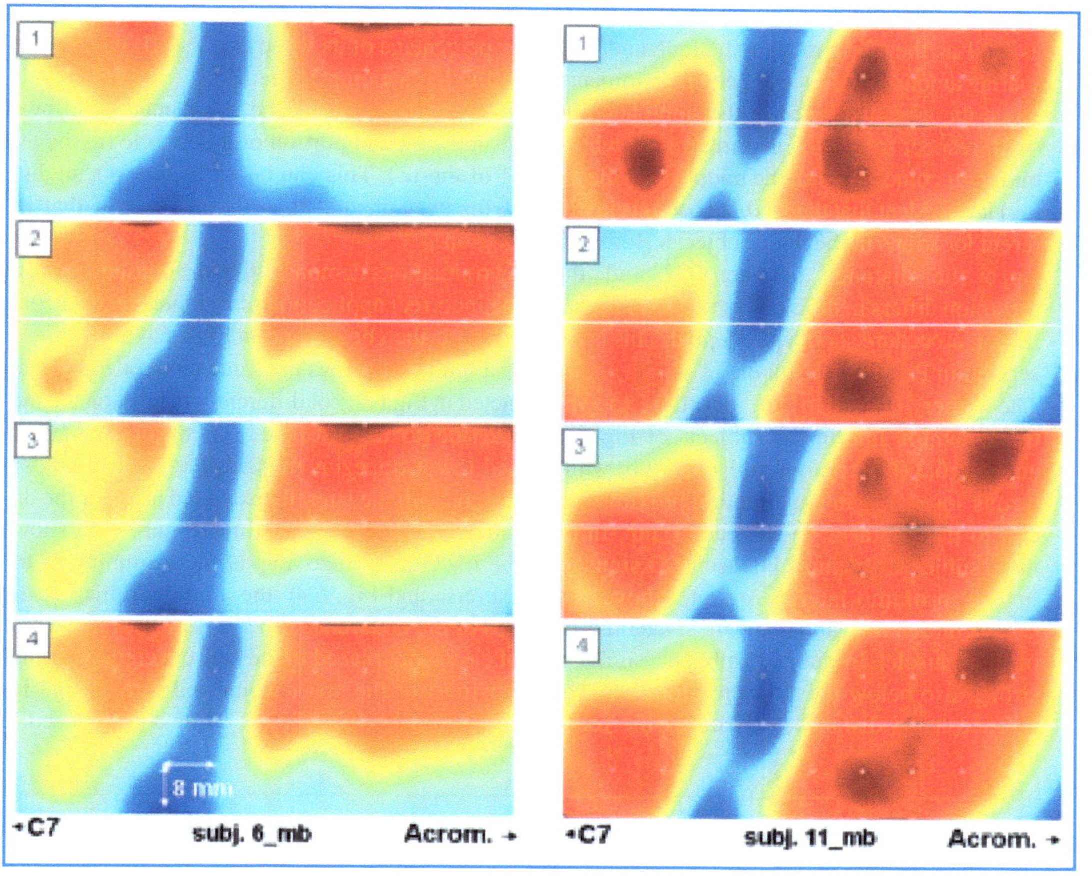


Fig. 6.3 Each vertical sequence of images represents four sequential interpolated ARV maps computed from LSD sEMG signals over 0.25 s epochs from the mid-upper trapezius of two subjects. The electrode arrangement and map orientation are the same as shown in Fig. 6.2a. The color scale is the same for the eight maps. Contraction level is 50% MVC. *White dots* indicate SD channels spaced 8 mm apart. *White line* C7–acromion line. Both subjects have a single IZ placed more medially than in the subject in Fig. 6.2. Minor differences from epoch to epoch are evident. Major differences between the subjects can also be readily appreciated (see also Fig. 6.2)

can be extracted with proper software) but the EMG-imaging technique of Fig. 6.2 gives an immediate perception of the muscle activity distribution on the skin, the location of the IZ, and the optimal location of a single pair of electrodes, which is obviously near the upper right corner of the array. At this point, we can also ask whether the EMG amplitude distribution on the trapezius muscle is the same for different individuals. In other words, are the IZ and the optimal location of a single electrode pair the same for different individuals? The answer requires a statistical investigation (see Part 2 of this book) and is hinted at by the maps depicted in Fig. 6.3.

Several observations can be made from the images shown in Figs. 6.2 and 6.3.

1. When the muscle depicted in Fig 6.2 increases its contraction level from 20% MVC to 80% MVC, the ARV map changes significantly in intensity (dark red corresponds to 80 μV at 20% MVC and to 260 μV at 80% MVC) but not much in shape, suggesting that the new MUs that are recruited when the force is increased have the same geometrical arrangements as those recruited at 20% MVC.
2. Small changes in the ARV distributions take place even within 1 s, but in Fig. 6.3 trends are barely visible. A longer observation time

(greater number of epochs) will evidence trends as well as the phenomena of fatigue and load sharing among muscles and their compartments.

3. Since the array is placed in the same position (with respect to the C7–acromion line, whose midpoint coincides with the midpoint of the array) it is evident that the IZ (blue band) is in different locations in the three subjects. However, since the distance between C7 and the acromion differs in different subjects, a normalization procedure should be adopted. This is described in Part 2 of this book.
4. The fiber direction is parallel to the C7–acromion line in the subjects of Fig. 6.2 and Fig. 6.3 (left column, subject 6_mb) while it runs somewhat in the direction proximo-lateral to medial-distal in subject 11_mb. In all three subjects, the most intense LSD signal is in the proximo-lateral region, above the C7–acromion line, and in the most lateral third of the muscle. In subj.11_mb, the signal is strong also below the C7–acromion line. The C7–acromion distance is taken as the reference and other distances are expressed as a percentage of its value (see Part II) when defining the location of the IZ.
5. In all three subjects, the signal intensity is lower in the medial portion of the muscle (to the left of the IZ). This can be attributed to a slightly thicker subcutaneous tissue layer in that region.

Two situations demonstrating the consequences of the incorrect application of a single electrode pair are described below and in Figs. 6.4 and 6.5.

Figure 6.4 shows the same electrode array depicted in Fig 6.2, but differently placed, on the medial side (to the left of the IZ) of the upper, median, and lower trapezius muscle. The subject holds a weight with the laterally extended arm, for the duration of the endurance time. Figure 6.4b shows the EMG amplitude map at the beginning of the exercise and Fig. 6.4c the amplitude map at the end of the endurance time. It is evident that a pair of electrodes placed in the area covered by the upper third of the array would indicate a large increase of EMG amplitude, while a pair placed in

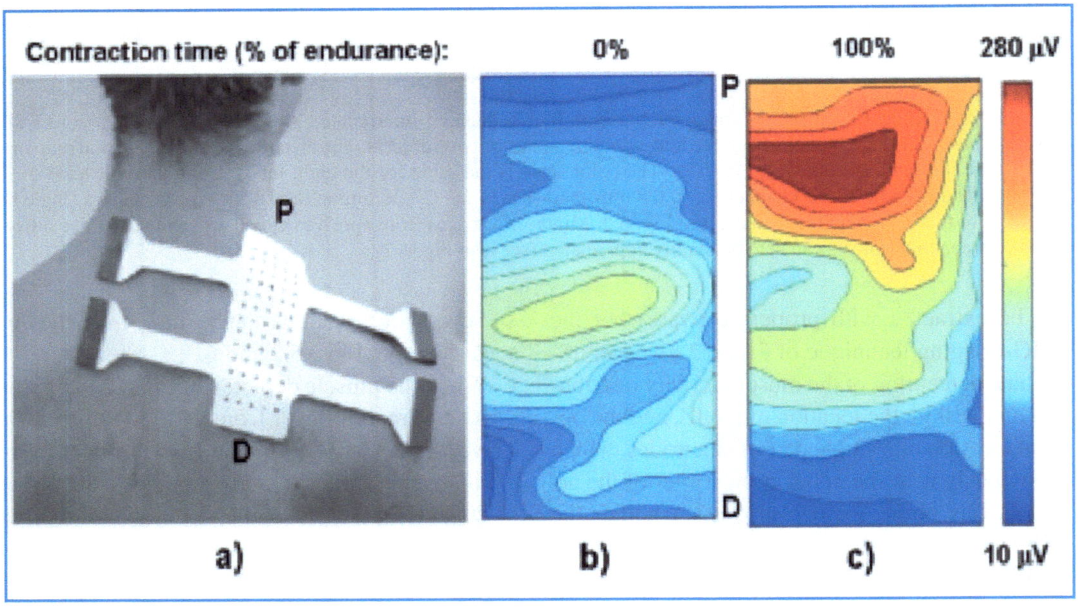


Fig. 6.4 A 5 × 13 contact electrode grid is placed on the trapezius muscle as indicated (a). The right arm is holding a weight and is horizontally extended laterally. The two interpolated maps show the EMG amplitude (ARV) at the beginning and at the end of an endurance experiment. It is clear which portion of the muscle is most active in the two conditions. A pair of electrodes placed over the green area would show no change between conditions b and c (reprinted from Farina et al., 2008)

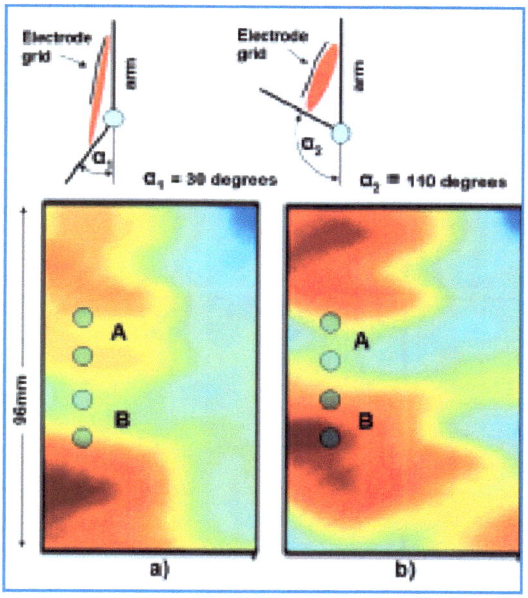


**Fig. 6.5** Interpolated image of the ARV of the LSD EMG detected from the biceps brachii with the array depicted in Fig. 6.4a. **a** Elbow almost fully extended; **b** forearm flexed 80°. The muscle shortens under the array, the IZ shifts upwards by 20–25 mm, and the distal tendon appears at the distal end of the array. Electrode pair A detects a decrease in the EMG amplitude, and electrode pair B an increase. Only the 2D image provides a description of what is happening. The IZ is an anatomical reference with respect to which a detection channel must maintain a fixed distance. This can be done with a linear or 2D electrode array, by defining a tracking criterion implemented on a computer with suitable software

the lower two thirds of the area covered by the array would indicate no significant change.

All the examples mentioned up to this point refer to isometric contractions, when the muscle undergoes minimal movements under the electrode array. The situation is very different in dynamic contractions, when the investigated muscle moves considerably underneath the array. Consider a 2D electrode array, such as that depicted in Fig. 6.2a, placed over the biceps brachii when the arm is extended. A contraction of the muscle produces the interpolated LSD sEMG amplitude map depicted in Fig. 6.5a. Suppose that the elbow joint slowly flexes by 80°. The muscle shortens under the array. The IZ moves proximally and the muscle-tendon junction appears under the distal end of the array (as indicated by the green area at the bottom of Fig. 6.5b). Consider what happens when one operator places a pair of electrodes in position A and another operator places another pair in position B. The first operator would claim that elbow flexion causes a decrease in the sEMG amplitude, and the second would provide evidence demonstrating the opposite. Indeed, what the two operators observe is a shortening of the biceps brachii and a shift of its IZ, which may reach 2–3 cm and slide from being under one electrode pair to being under the other, and *not necessarily* a change in the activity of the muscle. This is a very common mistake, induced by the statement, found in many books and manuals, that a pair of EMG electrodes should be placed "on the belly of the muscle," which is often the worst possible place because it frequently coincides with the location of the IZ. In a dynamic contraction, the electrodes should "move" with the muscle and their position should be related to the IZ rather than to a fixed anatomical reference. This can be done only by means of linear or 2D electrode arrays that allow tracking of the IZ and automatically choose the proper electrode pair or electrode group from the array.

Figure 6.6 shows an array of 128 electrodes applied on the gastrocnemius medialis and lateralis. Unlike the biceps brachii, the trapezius, and many other muscles, the gastrocnemius is pinnate, as indicated in Figs. 3.13–3.15; that is, its fibers are inclined with respect to the skin and connect two tendon layers called the aponeurosis. Neither the IZ nor the propagating APs are visible on the surface (see also Fig. 4.7) and the major contributions to the EMG are due to the end-of-fiber effect, described in Chapter 3, at the superficial aponeurosis (see Fig. 3.5).

Figures 6.2–6.6 show the possible differences in the sEMG amplitude maps for different muscles, given different conditions and array arrangements. Thus, EMG amplitude imaging provides a wealth of information that is still mostly untapped.

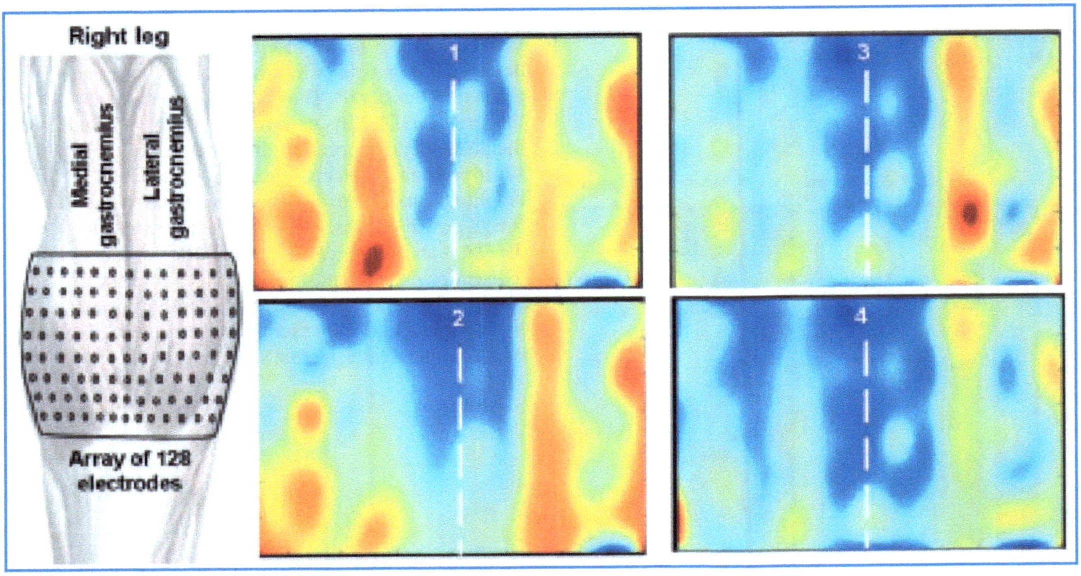


**Fig. 6.6** Four interpolated maps of sEMG amplitude (ARV) computed over four sequential epochs of 0.25 s, using a 128-electrode array covering the gastrocnemius medialis and lateralis during quiet standing. No IZ is detectable. During the observation time (1 s), the activity moves in space within each muscle and from one muscle to the other. Observe the difference with respect to the maps obtained from muscles with fibers parallel to the skin (Figs. 6.2 and 6.3). (Courtesy of T. Vieira)

## 6.2 Spectral Variables and Their Spatial Distribution

For each channel of a signal array and each time epoch (see Fig. 6.1), both amplitude variables (such as ARV or RMS) and spectral variables (such as MNF or MDF) can be computed. We can therefore have amplitude maps and "frequency" maps that change over time. For fusiform muscles with fibers parallel to the skin, as indicated in Fig. 5.7, the spectral variables of the SD sEMG signal are higher near the IZ because the signal is small, the noise generated at the electrode-skin junction becomes important, and the signal to noise ratio is lower. Since the noise spectrum is wider than the spectrum of the sEMG signal, the resulting MNF or MDF values will be higher. This is evident from Fig. 3.9, where channel 7, although much smaller than the other channels, has faster fluctuations due to the background noise. Near the endings of the fibers, the sharper end-of-fiber effect and the smaller signal to noise ratio also produce higher MND and MDF values. These phenomena are evident in 2D EMG frequency imaging. Figure 6.7 shows the interpolated distribution of MNF of the SD potential distribution under the electrode array depicted in Fig. 6.2.

The four maps depicted in Fig. 6.7 represent the interpolated spatial distribution of MNF (0.5 s epoch) at four points in time during the isometric sustained and constant-force (50% MVC) contraction of an upper trapezius muscle. Map 1 was recorded after 7 s of contraction, map 2 after 20 s, map 3 after 30 s, and map 4 after 40 s. The subject was able to sustain the contraction for 50 s.

The color scale represents the mean frequency values of the spectra of the single LSD channels. From the four images, we can observe the well-defined location of the IZ and the rather uniform distribution of MNF values to its right and left. We can also see that the decrement in the MNF over time is uniform in space and that no section of the muscle shows myoelectric manifestations of muscle fatigue greater than those of other sections. This is not always the case.

Figure 6.8 shows the initial and final ARV and MNF maps in another subject sustaining an isometric 50% MVC contraction of the upper trapezius to endurance. Each dot shown in Fig. 6.8a, b, e, and f indicates the ARV or MNF value relative

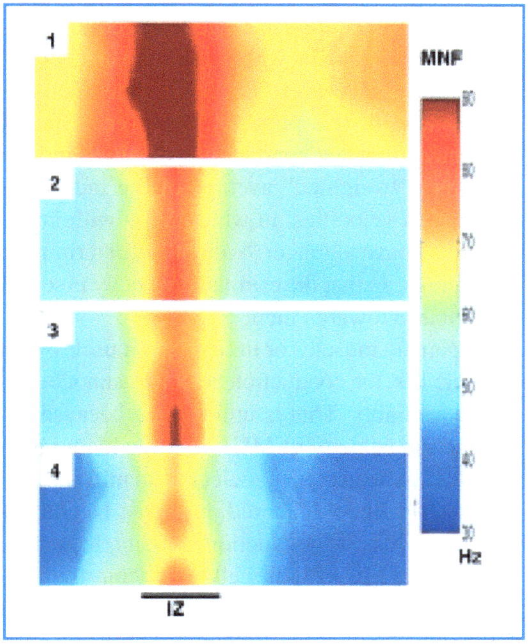


**Fig. 6.7** Example of the interpolated spatial distribution of MNF (0.5 s epoch, LSD signals) during the isometric and constant force (50% MVC) contraction of an upper trapezius muscle sustained to the endurance time (50 s). The four maps were obtained after 7, 20, 30, and 40 s, respectively. The color scale represents the MNF frequency values. A well-defined location of the IZ and the rather uniform distribution of MNF values to its right and its left can be observed. The position and features of the electrode array are indicated in Fig. 6.2. The progressively lower MNF values above the IZ are due to the progressively slower process of MUAP generation. In this case, the progressive decrement of MNF in time is uniform in space. It is evident that proper estimates of the MNF can be obtained from signals detected to the left and to the right of the IZ

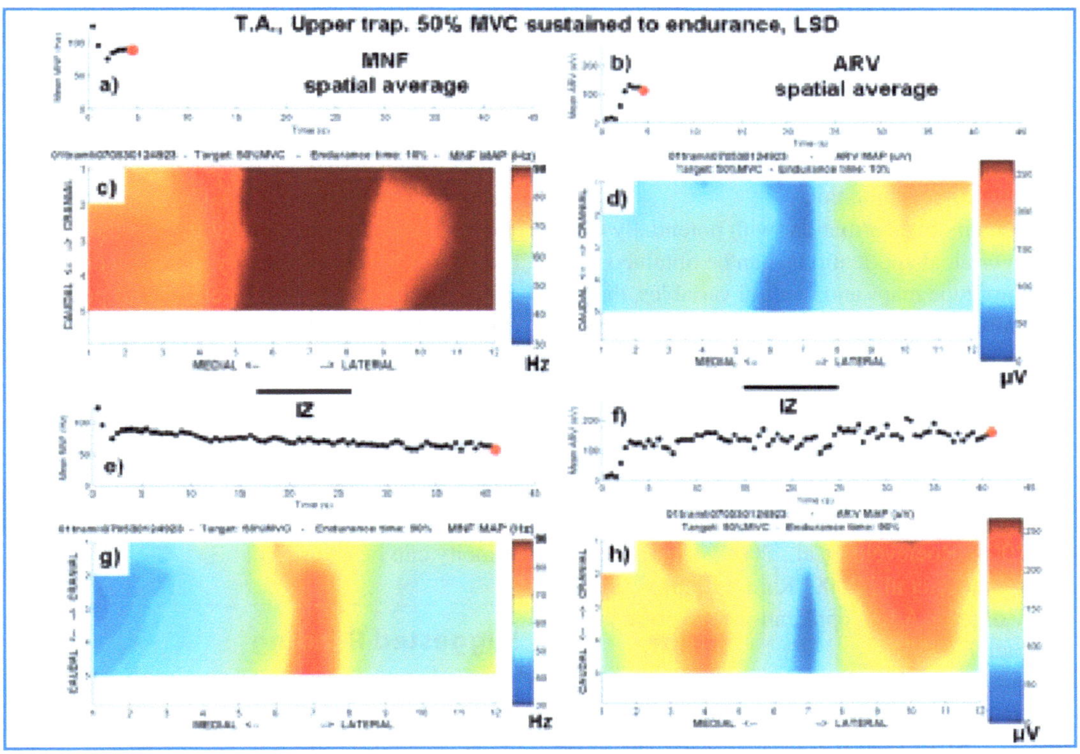


**Fig. 6.8** MNF and ARV maps during the isometric contraction of an upper trapezius muscle sustained to endurance at 50% MVC. LSD signals; epoch = 0.5 s. **a, b** Average in space of all the values of MNF and ARV computed every epoch up to the tenth epoch. **c, d** MNF and ARV maps after 5 s (tenth epoch). **e, f** Average in space of all the values of MNF and ARV computed every epoch. **g, h** MNF and ARV maps after 41 s (82nd epoch) at about 90% of the endurance time

to one epoch (0.5 s duration). This value is the result of the average in space of all the values (one for each LSD channel) obtained from the array for that epoch. While this representation may be very questionable, because it also includes the channels recorded over the IZ and the muscle-tendon junctions, it provides an indication of the *global* trend in space and time of the two variables.

Figure 6.8a, b identifies the eighth epoch, and Fig. 6.8c, d shows the MNF and ARV maps corresponding to that epoch. Figure 6.8e, f identifies one of the last epochs, a few seconds before the endurance time, and Fig. 6.8g, h the MNF and ARV maps corresponding to that epoch. The maps demonstrate how the spatial distribution of the MNF and ARV change as functions of time and provide information about the distribution of muscle activity in space and its evolution in time, as well as the distribution of myoelectric manifestations of fatigue in space and their evolution in time. On the basis of this information, either a properly trained human operator or computer software can select the most significant/representative area above a muscle and extract EMG features only from that area. In addition, the real-time presentation of this graphical information may provide new biofeedback techniques for training and rehabilitation.

Much more information (with potentially interesting clinical applications) can be obtained from the amplitude maps and spectral variables, that are currently being investigated in major research laboratories. Many of the applications of this information, ranging from the study of sports and cramps to that of neuromuscular disorders and ergonomics, have been reported in the literature (Farina and Merletti, 2000, 2002, 2004; Vieira et al., 2009; Merletti et al., 2009, 2010a, b; Minetto and Botter, 2009; Roeleveld et al., 2000; Minetto et al., 2010; Botter et al., 2009, Rainoldi, 2008; among many others). A few applications are presented in Chapter 7.

## 6.3 Spectral Variables and Muscle Fiber Conduction Velocity

The estimation of the conduction velocity of a single MUAP was described in Chapter 3 (Fig. 3.8). This procedure can be generalized to an interferential signal in which multiple MUs contribute their APs (Figs. 3.9, 3.10). Specific software exists for this purpose. However, different MUs have different conduction velocities and the result is a "weighted" average of the individual conduction velocities, in which MUs with larger potentials have a greater "weight" in determining the average, so that the estimated velocity is somewhat biased towards them.

In pinnate muscles or in fusiform muscles with multiple IZs, the conduction velocity cannot be estimated reliably. This is unfortunate because the conduction velocity of MUAPs is the main physiological indicator of myoelectric manifestations of muscle fatigue. It should, however, be considered that when the conduction velocity decreases, the detected MUAPs, as well as the contributions to the sEMG deriving from their generation and extinction processes, become wider (see Figs. 3.4, 3.6, 3.7). Consequently, the EMG spectrum becomes narrower (spectral compression) and the MNF and MDF decrease. Therefore, spectral variables reflect changes in conduction velocity and decrease everywhere when the conduction velocity decreases, although above the IZ their values are higher (see Figs. 6.7, 6.8). Unfortunately, spectral variables are affected by many other factors besides conduction velocity and reflect several different changes (of both central and peripheral origin) taking place in the muscle. Their interpretation accordingly requires great caution and is discussed in publications whose details are beyond the scope of this book (Mesin et al., 2009; Gallina et al., 2011). Despite these difficulties in interpretation, spectral variables are commonly regarded as indicators of fatigue whether or not conduction velocity can be estimated.

## Suggested Reading

Botter A, Lanfranco F, Merletti R, Minetto MA (2009) Myoelectric fatigue profiles of three knee extensor muscles. Int J Sports Med 30:408-417

Farina D, Leclerc F, Arendt-Nielsen L et al (2008) The change in spatial distribution of upper trapezius muscle activity is correlated to contraction duration J Electromyogr Kinesiol 18:16-25

Farina D, Cescon C, Merletti R (2002) Influence of anatomical, physical, and detection-system parameters on surface EMG. Biol Cybern 86:445-456

Farina D, Madeline P, Graven-Nielsen T et al (2002) Standardising surface electromyogram recordings for assessment of activity and fatigue in the human upper trapezius muscle. Eur J Appl Physiol 86:469-478

Farina D, Merletti R (2004) Methods for estimating muscle fibre conduction velocity from surface electromyographic signals. Med Biol Eng Comput 42:432-445

Farina D, Merletti R (2000) Comparison of algorithms for estimation of EMG variables during voluntary isometric contractions. J Electromyogr Kinesiol 10:337-349

Gallina A, Merletti R, Vieira TMM (2011) Are the myoelectric manifestations of fatigue distributed regionally in the human medial gastrocnemius muscle? J Electromyogr Kinesiol 21:928-938

Hedayatpour N, Arendt-Nielsen L, Farina D (2008) Non-uniform electromyographic activity during fatigue and recovery of the vastus medialis and lateralis muscles. J Electromyogr Kinesiol 18:390-396

Joseph J, Nightingale A, Williams PL (1955) A detailed study of the electric potentials recorded over some postural muscles while relaxed and standing. J Physiol 127:617-625

Merletti R, Aventaggiato M, Botter A et al (2010a) Advances in surface EMG: recent progress in detection and processing techniques. Crit Rev Biomed Eng 38:305-345

Merletti R, Botter A, Cescon C et al (2010b) Advances in surface EMG: recent progress in clinical research applications. Crit Rev Biomed Eng 38:347-379

Merletti R, Botter A, Troiano A et al (2009) Technology and instrumentation for detection and conditioning of the surface electromyographic signal: state of the art. Clin Biomech 24:122-134

Mesin L, Cescon C, Gazzoni M et al (2009) A bi-dimensional index for the selective assessment of myoelectric manifestations of peripheral and central muscle fatigue. J Electromyogr Kinesiol 19:851-863

Minetto MA, Botter A (2009) Elicitability of muscle cramps in different leg and foot muscles. Muscle Nerve 40:535-544

Minetto MA, Botter A, Lanfranco F et al (2010) Muscle fiber slowing and decreased levels of circulating muscle proteins after short term dexamethasone administration in healthy subjects. J Clin Endocr Metab 95:1663-1671

Rainoldi A, Falla D, Mellor R et al (2008) Myoelectric manifestations of fatigue in vastus lateralis, medialis obliquus and medialis longus muscles. J Electromyogr Kinesiol 18:1032-1037

Roeleveld K, van Engelen BG, Stegeman DF (2000) Possible mechanisms of muscle cramp from temporal and spatial surface EMG characteristics. J Appl Physiol 88:1698-1706

Tucker K, Falla D, Graven-Nielsen T, Farina D (2009) Electromyographic mapping of the erector spinae muscle with varying load and during sustained contraction. J Electromyogr Kinesiol 19:373-379

Vieira TMM, Merletti R, Farina D (2009) Intermittent recruitment of motor units in the medial gastrocnemius muscle during quiet standing. Gait Posture 30(Suppl 1):S17-18

# 7 Applications of sEMG in Dynamic Conditions, Ergonomics, Sports, and Obstetrics

**Abstract**

This book does not include a description of the criteria for the various sEMG applications nor does it define the clinical guidelines for their use. However, limited additional material and a few examples of applications are presented in this chapter, providing recommendations but also warnings. These examples have been selected among the many in which knowledge of the innervation zone of a muscle is relevant. Thus, it is essential that the operator pays great attention to the sEMG detection modalities to avoid reaching incorrect conclusions. Other applications concerning the use of maps of sEMG signals and of EMG variables for rehabilitation and the control of prosthesis, robots, etc., are not discussed; thus, the reader is referred to the many review articles on these topics listed in the reference section.

## 7.1 Why is it Important To Know the Location of the Innervation Zone?

Knowledge of the location of the IZ is important for the following reasons: (a) it allows correct estimation of the sEMG variables indicating the intensity of muscle electrical activity and muscle fatigue, in particular when a single electrode pair is used; (b) there are several interventions that require this knowledge (e.g., injection of botulinum toxin and episiotomy during child delivery). A summary of the basic concepts discussed in the previous chapters, and relevant to these topics is provided below.

When dealing with isometric contractions of fusiform muscles parallel to the skin, such as most of those listed in Part II of this book, there are several considerations:

1. A pair of electrodes placed over the IZ will register lower values of sEMG amplitude variables, such as ARV and RMS, which will more strongly depend on minor muscle or electrode displacements, as opposed to when both electrodes are positioned on one side of the IZ (see Figs. 3.12, 5.7, 6.8).
2. A pair of electrodes placed over the IZ will register higher values of sEMG spectral variables such as MNF and MDF, which will more strongly depend on minor muscle or electrode displacements, as opposed to when both electrodes are positioned on one side of the IZ (Figs. 5.7, 6.8).
3. In estimations of muscle fiber conduction velocity, the electrode array used for this purpose must be placed on one side of the IZ, or only channels on one side of the IZ must be selected to estimate conduction velocity (Fig. 3.8).
4. In dynamic conditions, the operator must be aware that any relative sliding between electrodes and the IZ during the movement may significantly modify all sEMG variables, possibly leading to misinterpretation of the results (Figs. 3.11, 3.12, 6.5).

In general, in pinnate muscles these considerations do not apply, or they are less relevant, except in regions near the end of certain muscles (such as the gastrocnemius), where the fibers are not covered by the muscle-tendon junctions of other fibers (Figs. 3.15, 4.7).

The main research topics in the sEMG field that remain under active investigation concern: (a) using the displacement of the IZ to estimate muscle shortening or lengthening, since the IZ provides an anatomical marker of the muscle; (b) identifying regions above the muscle from which changes in the sEMG can be reasonably associated with changes in muscle neural drive or force and not with geometrical factors; (c) estimating the relevance of cross-talk from nearby muscles, (Martin and Mac Isaac, 2006; Rainoldi et al., 2000; Mesin et al., 2009); (d) estimating the contributions of individual muscles to the total force or torque acting at the joint (Merletti et al., 2010a, b; Karlsson et al., 2009; Staudeman et al., 2009).

## 7.2 Applications in Dynamic Conditions

Dynamic conditions in fusiform muscles parallel to the skin are very difficult to study with only one pair of electrodes because any observed change in sEMG variables may be due either to a change in muscle activation level or to a change in the geometry of the electrode-muscle system. To discriminate between these two possible interpretations, a linear electrode array (Fig. 3.11) or, and better, a 2D array (Fig. 6.5) is required. Active regions can then be selected, such as the darkest red regions in Fig 6.5, and should be identified and tracked, possibly on-line, as the muscle moves under the electrodes. Surface EMG variables should then be identified from a subset of electrodes that change during movement. Tracking the moving IZ and segmentation of the image into the moving regions of interest become very important in these cases. Recent research has addressed these issues (Zwarts and Stegeman, 2003; Farina, 2006; Drost et al., 2006; Karlsson et al., 2009; Staudeman et al., 2009; Merletti et al., 2010a, b).

If only one pair of electrodes is to be used, its position must be defined after a few tests in order to be reasonably sure that it detects a signal generated by the same muscle portion. Since this may not always be possible, bipolar sEMG recordings in dynamic conditions must be considered with great caution because the sEMG variables may reflect geometrical changes rather than changes in muscle activation levels. (Farina et al., 2004; Farina, 2006).

In highly dynamic conditions, such as cycling, repeated jumping, and fast elbow flexion-extensions, a stroboscopic analysis may be applied to select time epochs that correspond to the same muscle position in subsequent repetitions of the periodic task (Bonato et al., 2001; Macdonald et al., 2008).

Experience concerning pinnate muscles in dynamic conditions is limited. The electrodes on the skin read mostly the end-of-fiber effect of the motor units (MUs) terminating below the electrodes, at the superficial aponeurosis (Figs. 3.13–3.15). The territory of such MUs may be localized or scattered, as may be their activity (Fig. 6.6). In addition, the pinnation angle changes with the produced force and with the joint angle due to the elasticity of the tendons. *Accordingly, a local change in amplitude of the sEMG, as detected by a single electrode pair, does not necessarily imply or prove a change in the muscle activation level.* This is particularly the case in fusiform muscles when the electrode pair is placed over or near the IZ.

## 7.3 Applications in Ergonomics

Ergonomics is a very important area of sEMG application. Some muscles involved in joint stabilization during a working task operate in nearly isometric conditions (e.g., the trapezius, back muscles), a fact that simplifies the task of monitoring their activity. Work-related musculoskeletal disorders of the neck-shoulder region are a social and economic problem in Western society and the risk of developing shoulder and neck pain is particularly pronounced in those whose work involves long hours on the computer (Goudy and McLean, 2006; Christensen and Sjøgaard, 1999; Sandsjö and Kadefors, 2001).

The examples presented in this section are limited to the trapezius muscle but other muscles of the upper limb have been investigated (Rainoldi et al., 2008; Bonfiglioli et al., 2012). Figures 6.2–6.4

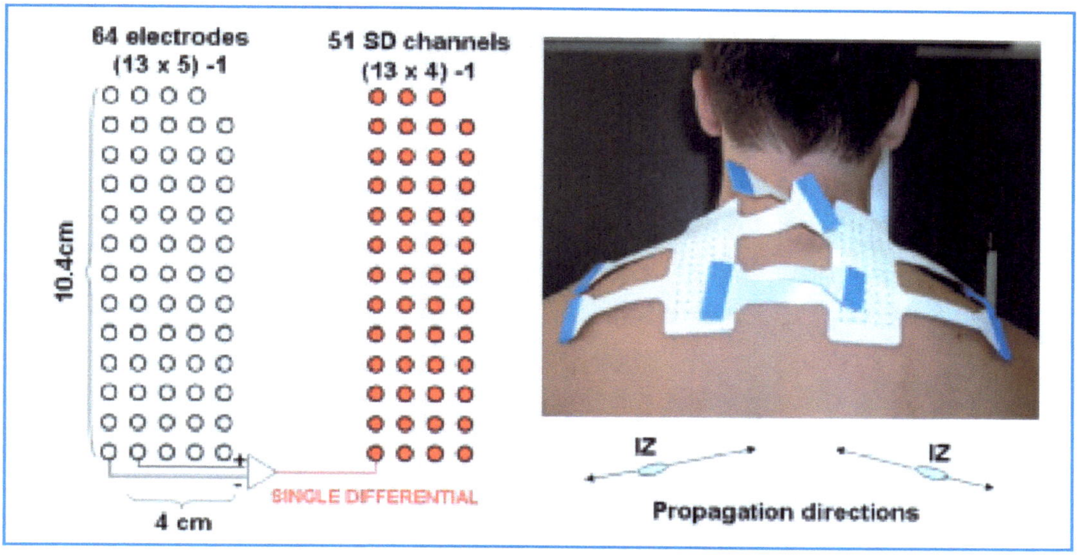


**Fig. 7.1** Example of an application in which two 2D electrode arrays are placed on the upper and middle trapezius, medially with respect to the IZ, with rows in the direction of the fibers. Single differential sEMG signals are computed in the fiber direction (LSD); a map of the ARV values is obtained over 30 s of computer activity and then interpolated. Three postures are considered and associated with sEMG activity. The results are reported in Figs. 7.2 and 7.3. The subject is right-handed. (Courtesy of A. Gallina)

show a 2D array placed above the trapezius muscle during isometric constant-force contractions. The array is placed in two different ways, covering the entire upper trapezius or the medial portions of the upper and middle trapezius, with either columns or rows approximately aligned with the direction of the muscle fibers.

Figure 7.1 shows the arrangement of two 2D arrays placed, as in Fig. 6.4, on the medial side of the IZ of the upper and middle trapezius muscle, with rows in the direction of the fibers and differential sEMG signals computed along the rows. The ARV maps of the sEMG LSD signals are displayed in Figs. 7.2 and 7.3 and can be used to investigate activation of the trapezius in a computer user working with keyboard and mouse. Different distributions and levels of activity can be observed depending on the position of the arms (wrist support, forearm support, no support).

The relevance of properly detected sEMG signals in assessing the best occupational set-ups or in monitoring a worker's activity is evident. The images provided in Figs. 7.2 and 7.3 can be used either to improve the workstation or to teach the operator the correct posture to avoid muscle hyperactivities possibly resulting in eventual muscle stress, inflammation, or pain (Gazzoni, 2010).

## 7.4 Applications in Exercise and Sports

This section provides tutorial examples of experimental protocols and results concerning sEMG applications in sports, in which proper electrode positioning is critical (Rainoldi et al., 2000). Figure 7.4a shows a 2D electrode array (128 electrodes) applied above the vastus medialis muscle of a subject performing an isometric effort of knee extension, and Fig. 7.4b the amplitude map of LSD signals computed in the approximate direction of the muscle fibers (45°, along the dashed line of Fig. 7.4a, b; this is not the direction along the columns of the array). The blue regions identify the IZ and the muscle-tendon junctions of the muscle; the red regions are those of high signal amplitude. If the knee moves (dynamic contraction), a short electrode array, or an electrode pair, must remain in one of the red regions to assure that geometrical effects on the recorded sEMG ampli-

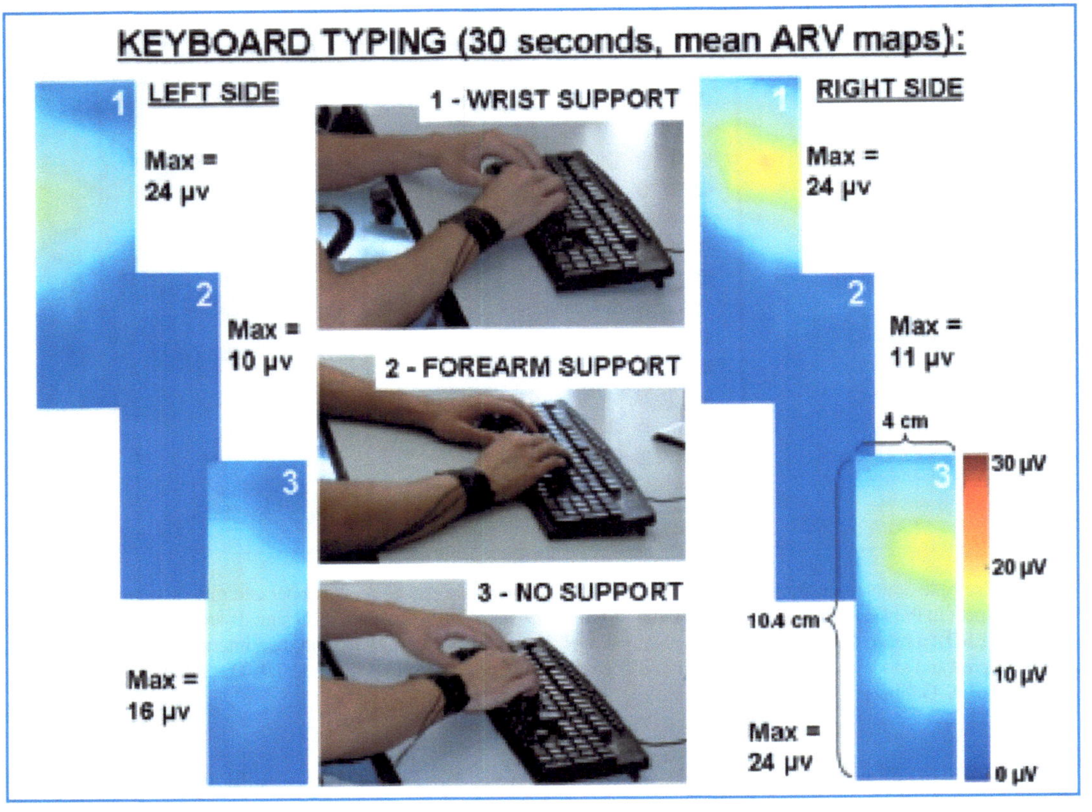


**Fig. 7.2** The sEMG maps obtained from the electrode arrangements described in Fig. 7.1, while the subject types on a keyboard. *Case 1*: the chair is low and only the wrists are in contact with the desk. *Case 2*: the chair has the correct height and the forearms are resting on the desk. The keyboard is away from the edge of the desk. *Case 3*: the chair is too high and the forearms are not in contact with the desk. Only in case 2 is trapezius activity near zero. In cases 1 and 3, activity is present predominantly in the right upper trapezius. Color scales are the same for all maps. (Courtesy of A. Gallina)

tude are minimized (see Fig. 6.4 for the case of the biceps brachii). If this condition is not met, the conclusions obtained from the experiments will very likely be incorrect.

Examples of three experimental protocols are shown below. Great care was invested in identifying electrode positions suitable to avoid geometrical effects and to outline different degrees of myoelectric manifestations of muscle fatigue and muscle activation in different conditions.

**Example 1.** A specific protocol was designed to highlight the effect of oxygen availability in endurance and power trained athletes. Oxygen availability to a muscle is one of the pivotal factors affecting muscle fatigue (Casale et al., 2004) and is reduced in ischemic muscles, specifically during sustained medium-high contractions because of the high intramuscular pressure. Mechanical performance was not significantly altered when endurance or power athletes switched from intermittent (1 s of rest between contractions) to continuous (same force level but without breaks) contractions, as indicated in Fig. 7.5a. However, the rate of decrement of muscle fiber conduction velocity (a classical fatigue index) increased significantly (see Fig. 7.5b) in endurance-trained athletes whereas in power-trained athletes it was not modified (Rainoldi et al., 2010) by the introduction of short breaks. This approach demonstrates the sensitivity of sEMG parameters to different contraction modalities and phenotypes. Its use has been proposed as a non-invasive technique to distinguish between the two phenotypes.

**Example 2**. A recent study compared the role

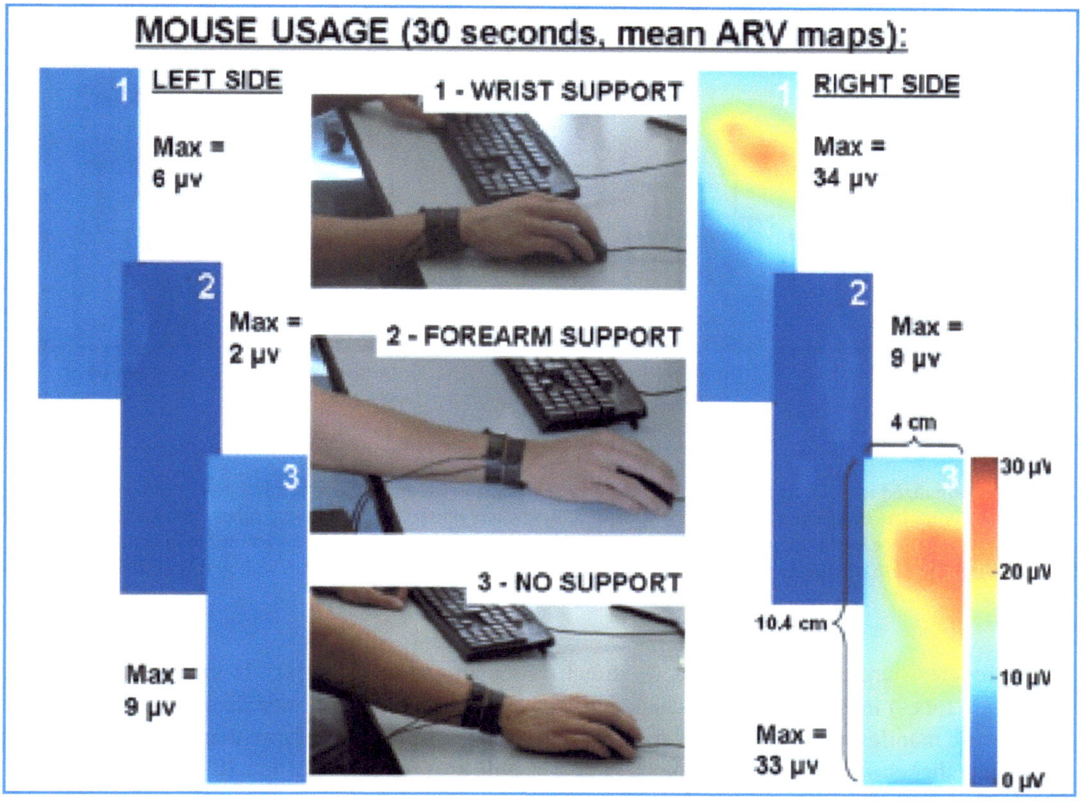


**Fig. 7.3** EMG maps obtained from the electrode arrangements described in Fig. 7.1, while the subject uses a mouse. *Case 1*: the chair is low and only the wrist is in contact with the desk. *Case 2*: the chair has the proper height and the forearms are resting on the desk. *Case 3*: the chair is high and the forearms are not in contact with the desk. Only in case 2 is trapezius activity near zero. In cases 1 and 3, activity is present and strongly predominant in the right upper trapezius, with some involvement of the middle trapezius in case 3. (Courtesy of A. Gallina)

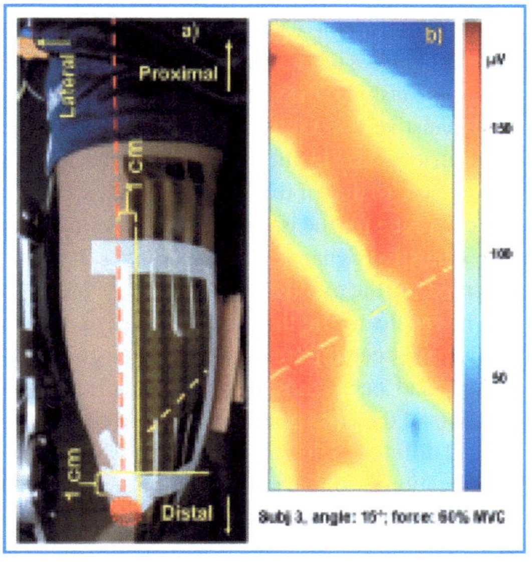


**Fig. 7.4** **a** The surface 2D electrode array is placed above the vastus medialis muscle of the right leg of a subject. The knee angle is 15° (0° is full extension) and force is 60% MVC. IED = 10 mm. Single differential EMG signals are computed along a direction at 45°, close to the fiber direction (*dashed yellow line*). **b** Interpolated amplitude map of the single differential EMG signals clearly showing areas of high (*red*) and low (*blue*) amplitude. The IZ is readily visible in the middle. Short arrays or single electrode pairs must be placed in the red area and remain there if (during dynamic contractions) the knee angle changes

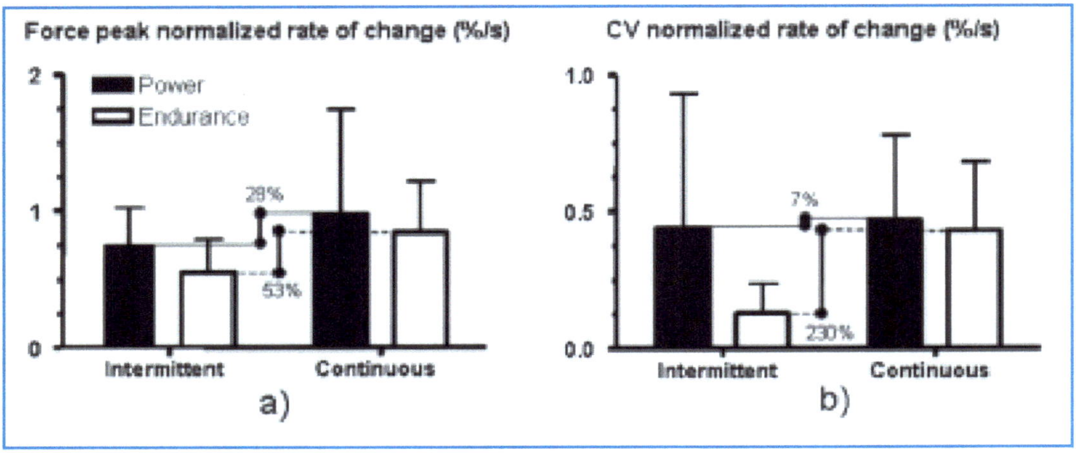


**Fig. 7.5** Normalized rates of change of force peak of knee extension (**a**) and conduction velocity (**b**) in continuous and intermittent contractions performed by two groups of athletes, one power-trained and the other endurance-trained. The increment of the myoelectric fatigue index in continuous vs. intermittent contraction was greater in the latter group. The mean ± SD of the rate of change of force and conduction velocity is reported (reprinted with permission from Rainoldi and Gazzoni, 2010)

of different resistances (lifting weights vs. stretching elastic tubes) in determining mechanical and myoelectric manifestations of fatigue, specifically asking whether elastic exercise determined greater fatigue than traditional exercise, based on a standardized isometric contraction performed immediately after a training section (Melchiorri and Rainoldi, 2011). The findings confirmed that contractions achieved with the use of elastic bands require greater muscle activation; moreover, they highlight a sort of "muscle conditioning" after the specific contraction modality that requires the use of faster MUs. It is thus possible to consider the practical use of such elastic devices to increase neuromuscular activation, for instance in specific rehabilitation settings in which slow movements with minimal risk of injury are desired (post-surgery rehabilitation, physical activity by the elderly or by children).

**Example 3.** A highly dynamic exercise was used to compare the activities of the brachioradialis and teres major muscles in climbers performing three different pull-up tasks on a special board used to strengthen the arms and forearms in a sport-specific manner (Formicola et al., 2010). The first task consisted of an isometric contraction until exhaustion in order to maintain the body hanging with a finger grip, the elbow flexed at 90°, and the arm abducted at 90°. In the second task, five pull-ups were performed as fast as possible. The third task was to perform an unlimited number of pull-ups, until exhaustion (END). An electrogoniometer placed on the elbow, used as trigger, allowed identification of the eccentric and concentric phases. The following was observed: (1) sEMG amplitudes were higher in the concentric phases (presumably reflecting higher MU recruitment and discharge rates) than in the eccentric phases; (2) explosive tasks were not associated with higher activation (in terms of global sEMG variables) but with higher rates of fatigue than determined for the exhaustive task; (3) the sEMG amplitude in isometric exhaustive contraction was lower than in the concentric phase in the two dynamic tasks, but comparable to that of the eccentric phases; (4) the rate of fatigue for the isometric task was similar to the exhaustive dynamic task, and lower than that observed for the explosive task.

The results of the three examples given above would have been different if different electrode locations had been chosen, or if the selection of channels of the array to be used for EMG processing had differed. Selecting the correct EMG detection location is of paramount importance in the sEMG analysis of physical exercise and sport activities.

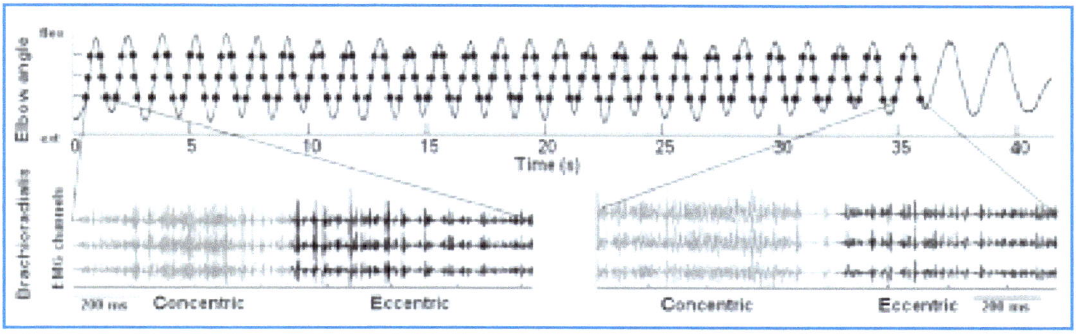


Fig. 7.6 Signals recorded during the "END" task described in Example 3 (see text). The top trace shows the time course of the elbow angle during the endurance exercise. *Black dots* identify the center of the 125 ms time intervals during which the EMG variables were estimated (crossing of 25%, 50%, and 75% of the elbow angle range). On the bottom, the double differential EMG signals recorded from the brachioradialis muscle during the first (*left*) and last (*right*) contractions are shown. The concentric and eccentric phases are plotted in *light gray* and *black*, respectively

## 7.5 Applications in Obstetrics

Episiotomy is a minor surgery frequently performed during natural child delivery to prevent tears of the vaginal wall. A pair of scissors is used to cut the vaginal wall, usually to the right (because most operators are right handed), in a direction tangential to the external anal sphincter (EAS). This cut is then sutured with a few stitches after passage of the child through the birth canal.

Tissue wounds that occur during natural childbirth (spontaneous tears or episiotomy) are significantly correlated with the subsequent appearance of fecal incontinence in women (Wheeler and Richter, 2007). However, given the very large intersubject variability in the location of the IZs of the EAS (Enck et al., 2004, Merletti et al., 2004), it is impossible to provide general guidelines that would allow episiotomies to be performed such that the EAS and its innervation are spared.

However, electromyography of the EAS can be performed by means of a cylindrical probe with an array of 16 electrodes equally spaced along the circumference of the probe. The procedure allows identification of the IZs of this muscle in individual subjects (Merletti et al., 2004), as indicated in Fig. 7.7.

In pregnant women, determining the location of the IZs of the anal sphincter would allow their avoidance in case episiotomy is deemed necessary at the time of delivery. This would lead to a significant reduction in the complications of this type of surgery. Figure 7.8 provides an example of the dependency of the risk of this surgical incision on the number and location of EAS innervation zones.

## 7.6 Other Applications and Future Perspectives

In many other sEMG applications, the use of sEMG maps is required to identify the correct electrode locations or the correct set of channels from an array designed for a specific purpose. These rapidly developing applications range from the study of masticatory muscles to the identification of the most effective site for the injection of botulinum toxin into spastic muscles. Biofeedback applications of sEMG amplitude maps provide new rehabilitation modalities to teach patients to activate a specific muscle or group of muscles by controlling the color pattern of the displayed map. A subset of channels selected from an electrode array could be used to control exoskeletons or games or even to generate music either for entertainment or rehabilitation.

Other new and interesting fields concern the use of sEMG for the control of remote devices and robots, specifically of "rehabilitation robots", able to use an EMG map to verify and adjust the actions they are performing on a patient.

We can imagine sleeves or garments carrying hundreds of electrodes covering an entire limb,

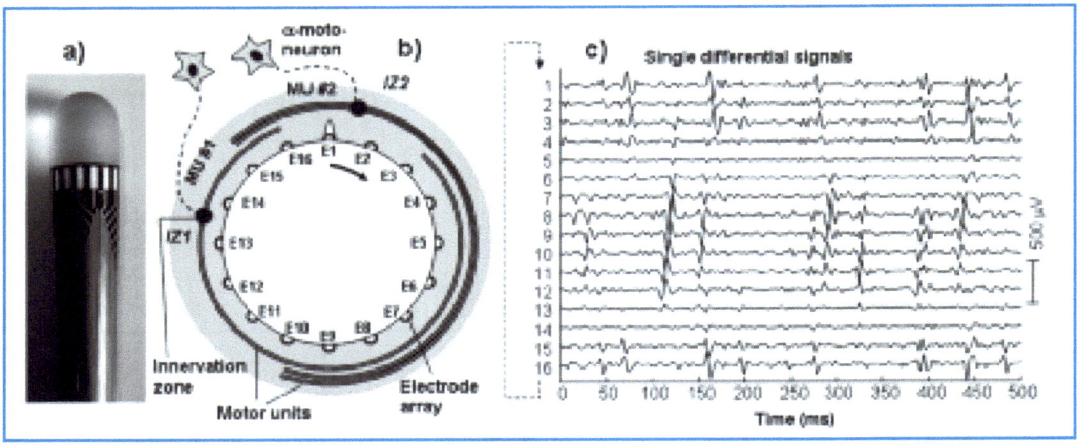


**Fig. 7.7** **a** Example of an intra-anal probe (diameter =14 mm) with 16 electrodes equally spaced around the circumference. **b** Schematic drawing of the electrode array and two MUs innervated in different locations. **c** Example of a 16 channel single differential recording during a voluntary contraction of the sphincter. Note that in this circular configuration electrode 16 is next to electrode 1 (therefore there are 16 single differential EMG channels). Also note that MUs are not innervated in their central region but often near one end and that propagation is unidirectional. Many MUs in this example are innervated under channels 13–14

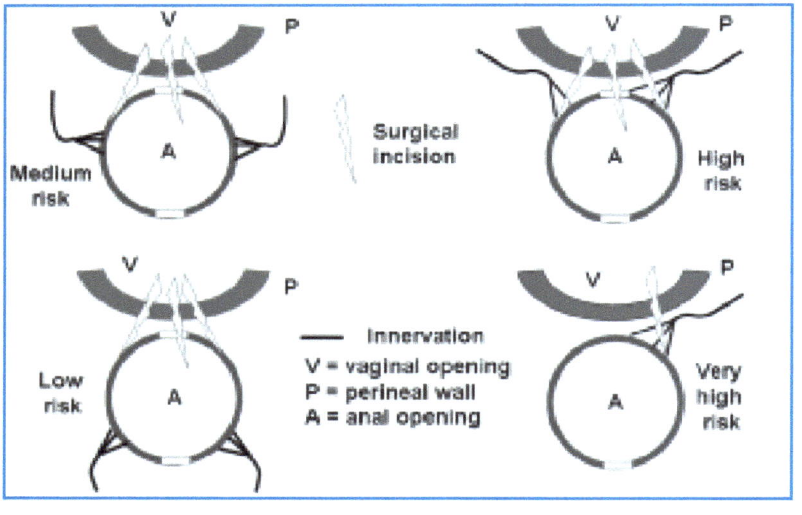


**Fig. 7.8** Schematic drawing of the vaginal (*V*) and anal (*A*) canals and of the four innervation patterns of the external anal sphincter (EAS), corresponding to four different levels of risk associated with episiotomy (surgical incision)

the entire trunk, or even most of the body, incorporating "intelligent" electronic systems that automatically replace "bad channels" (electrodes with poor contacts or high interferences), select regions of trustworthy signals, and transmit this information through a wireless link to a nearby computer or to the internet, via an access point, where the information of interest is extracted and processed for the desired purpose. Such techniques and devices can be expected in the near future.

## Suggested Reading

Bonato P, Roy SH, Knaflitz M, De Luca CJ (2001) Time-frequency parameters of the surface myoelectric signal for assessing muscle fatigue during cyclic dynamic contractions. IEEE Trans Biomed Eng 48:745-753

Bonfiglioli R, Botter A, Calabrese M et al (2012) Muscle nerve (in press doi:10.1002/mus.23258)

Casale R, Farina D, Merletti R, Rainoldi A (2004) Myoelectric manifestations of fatigue during exposure to hypobaric hypoxia for 12 days. Muscle Nerve 30:618-625

Christensen H, Sjøgaard G (1999) Symposium on muscular disorders in computer users: mechanisms and models. National Institute of Occupational Health, Copenhagen

Drost G, Stegeman DF, van Engelen BG, Zwarts MJ (2006) Clinical applications of high-density surface EMG: a systematic review. J Electromyogr Kinesiol 16:586-602

Enck P, Franz H, Azpiroz F et al (2004) Innervation zones of the external anal sphincter in healthy male and female subjects. Preliminary results. Digestion 69:123-130

Farina D, Pozzo M, Merlo E et al (2004) Assessment of average muscle fiber conduction velocity from surface EMG signals during fatiguing dynamic contractions. IEEE Trans Biomed Eng 51:1383-1393

Farina D (2006) Interpretation of the surface electromyogram in dynamic contractions. Exerc Sport Sci Rev 34:121-127

Formicola D, Gazzoni M, Pizzigalli L et al (2010) Neuromechanical characterization of two different techniques of rock climbing, Proceedings of ISEK 2010, Aalborg, Denmark DK

Gazzoni M (2010) Multi-channel surface EMG in ergonomics: potentialities and limits. Human Factors and Ergonomics in Manufacturing 20:255–271

Goudy N, McLean L (2006) Using myoelectric signal parameters to distinguish between computer workers with and without trapezius myalgia. Eur J Appl Physiol 97:196-209

Karlsson S, Roeleveld K, Gronlund C et al (2009) Signal processing of the surface electromyogram to gain insight into neuromuscular physiology. Philos Transact A Math Phys Eng Sci 367:337-356

Macdonald JH, Farina D, Marcora SM (2008) Response of electromyographic variables during incremental and fatiguing cycling. Med Sci Sports Exerc 40:335-344

Martin S, Mac Isaac D (2006) Innervation zone shift with changes in joint angle in the brachial biceps. J Electromyogr Kinesiol 16:144-148

Melchiorri G, Rainoldi A (2011) Muscle fatigue induced by two different resistances: Elastic tubing versus weight machines. J Electromyogr Kinesiol 21:954-959

Merletti R, Aventaggiato M, Botter A et al (2010a) Advances in surface EMG: recent progress in detection and processing techniques. Crit Rev Biomed Eng 38:305-345

Merletti R, Botter A, Cescon C et al (2010b) Advances in surface EMG: recent progress in clinical research applications. Crit Rev Biomed Eng 38:347-379

Merletti R, Bottin A, Cescon C et al (2004) Multichannel surface EMG for non invasive assessment of the anal sphincter muscle. Digestion 69:112-122

Mesin L, Smith S, Hugo S et al (2009) Effect of spatial filtering on crosstalk reduction in surface EMG recordings. Med Eng Phys 31:374-383

Rainoldi A, Nazzaro M, Merletti R et al (2000) Geometrical factors in surface EMG of the vastus medialis and lateralis. J Electromyogr Kinesiol 10:327-336

Rainoldi A, Gazzoni M (2010) Neuromuscular physiology. In: Cardinale M, Newton R, Nosaka K (eds) Strength and conditioning: biological principles and practical applications. Wiley, Chichester, UK

Rainoldi A, Bergamo R, Merlo A (2008) Atlas of the innervation zones of the superficial muscles of the shoulder. In: Fusco A, Foglia A, Musarra F, Testa M (eds) The shoulder in sport. Churchill Livingstone, Elsevier, Oxford, UK

Sandsjö L, Kadefors R (2001) Symposium on muscle disorders in computer users: scientific basis and recommendations. National Institute for Working Life, Göteborg

Staudenmann D, Roeleveld K, Stegeman DF, van Dieën JH (2009) Methodological aspects of SEMG recordings for force estimation: a tutorial and review. J Electromyogr Kinesiol 20:375-387

Wheeler TL, Richter HE (2007) Delivery method, anal sphincter tears and fecal incontinence: new information on a persistent problem. Curr Opin Obstet Gynecol 19:474-479

Zwarts MJ, Stegeman DF (2003) Multichannel surface EMG: basic aspects and clinical utility. Muscle Nerve 28:1-17

# Part II

*Marco Barbero*
*and Alberto Rainoldi*

## General Remarks

The theoretical approach described in Part I of this book provides the reader with useful information on three important issues: (1) how to record and analyze sEMG signals, (2) what information can be extracted from these signals, and (3) how this information should be interpreted. Until relatively recently, a detailed processing and interpretation of sEMG signals was deemed unnecessary due to the lack of awareness of the influence of electrode location on the quality and quantity of the obtainable information. As is often (if not always) the case, technological evolution provided new tools that increased our capability to understand issues related to volume conduction, the location of innervation zones, motor-unit recruitment strategies, etc.

In particular, the innervation zone (IZ) of a fusiform muscle parallel to the skin has now been clearly identified as the worst site to place a pair of recording electrodes. This area (often incorrectly called the neuromuscular junction or motor end plate) is the physical region where the central ($\alpha$-motor neuron terminations) and peripheral (muscle fibers) systems connect through special synapses: the neuromuscular junctions, or end plates. From each of these junctions, action potentials travel in opposite directions, toward the tendon terminations, and generate propagating potentials on the skin. As described in Part I, this issue is not relevant to pinnate muscles, as their fibers are not parallel to the skin.

According to a naive earlier approach, electrodes were placed in the middle of the muscle, over its bulk (or belly), since that zone is not only easy to identify by palpation but it also offers the greatest amount of muscle volume, corresponding (presumably!) to the largest EMG signal. This is a good example of an incorrect syllogism. Since the most common electrode montage is differential, it is clear that, if the IZ falls underneath the electrode pair, the resulting signal will be very small and noisy and highly affected by small electrode displacements. Indeed, in this case, signals generated by action potentials traveling toward one tendon are subtracted from similar signals generated by action potentials traveling in the opposite direction, with a resulting output that is small and noisy and often close to zero. Moreover, during dynamic contractions, the relative movement of the muscle with respect to the skin (that is the electrode system) determines a strong alteration of the signal when the IZ shifts under the electrode pair.

Now imagine a situation in which the effectiveness of treatment is being assessed based on a comparison of sEMG signals before and after an intervention. Consider electrodes placed over the IZ before the intervention and in a more correct location (which could be less than a couple of centimeters away along the fiber direction) after the intervention. Should the increased signal amplitude be attributed to the treatment or to altered electrode positioning? And what would the practitioner's conclusions be if the electrodes were placed properly before and wrongly after the treatment?

This important confounding factor cannot be ignored. Practitioners are interested in using sEMG to obtain information about muscle activation and timing during movements and to compare muscle activity before and after treatments, surgery, trainings, etc. In all such cases, the electrodes must be properly placed to avoid the incorrect and misleading conclusions discussed in Part I, for example in Fig. 6.5.

Since, for the moment, high-density EMG recording techniques are available almost exclusively in research laboratories, this Atlas provides practitioners with guidelines to find the best electrode placement on the most superficial muscles.

## Interpretation of the Charts and Plots

Surface EMG signals were recorded, during isometric contractions, from 43 muscles of 40 subjects (20 male and 20 female) and the "quality" of the signals from each muscle (good, fair, poor) was assessed on the basis of: (a) the quality of the recordable signals (presence of noise and interferences), (b) the observability of IZ(s), (c) the presence of signals propagating with physiological values of muscle-fiber conduction velocity (2–8 m/s), (d) the availability of an area large enough for a standard electrode pair (2–3 cm). The information is provided in the tables describing each muscle, together with a sample of the recorded signals, an anatomical sketch of the investigated muscle, and the distribution of the observed IZ regions in the 40 subjects, as described with "box and whiskers" plots. These plots show the distribution of the IZs in those subjects and muscles where they could be identified, the median location (half of the observations on one side and half on the other side of the median), the lower quartile (25% of the observations below and 75% above), the upper quartile (75% of the observations below and 25% above), and the minimum and maximum observations.

For each muscle, an anatomical landmark frame (ALF) was defined and is reported in the table, thus allowing the user to properly and univocally locate the area reported in the graph.

Hence, this Atlas suggests where the electrodes should *not* be placed. Since the best placement for bipolar electrode recording is the muscle area between the IZ and the distal/proximal tendon, the operator can determine proper electrode placement by following the anatomical landmarks provided in Part II, avoiding the shaded red areas and, possibly, the "whiskers."

## Interpretation of Muscle- and Signal-Quality Assessments

The "quality" of each muscle was assessed using a multi-criteria approach aimed at providing the reader with score-like information, as obtained with a set of hierarchical criteria. Very important criteria are weighted 2 points if met and 0 points if not met. Important criteria are weighted 0 points or 1 point.

### Criterion 1: Signal Quality (Score: 0 or 2 Points)

Is it possible to easily record the signal without noise? This is of course pivotal for further analysis.

### Criterion 2: Region Free From Innervation Zones (Score: 0 or 2 Points)

Is there a region long enough (> 20 mm) to place two electrodes far from the IZ?

### Criterion 3: Visual Detectability of the Propagation (Score: 0 or 1 Points)

Do recorded action potentials show physiological propagation (at a speed of 2–8 m/s) or does the signal mostly comprise non-traveling components? That is, is it possible to properly estimate conduction velocity? This issue is important for further advanced analysis, for instance, to estimate myoelectric manifestations of fatigue, but it is not crucial, for instance, to monitor muscle activation intervals.

### Crierion 4: Detectability of Motor Units (Score: 0 or 1 Points)

Is it possible to clearly recognize individual motor units and then classify them? As for criterion 3, this is important for advanced analysis but is not the goal of most practitioners.

| Signal quality analysis | |
|---|---|
| **Criteria** | **Points** |
| Signal quality (signal above the noise level) | 0 or 2 |
| Area free from IZ | 0 or 2 |
| Physiological signal propagation | 0 or 1 |
| Motor-units identification | 0 or 1 |

## Analyis of Recorded Signals

Figures II-1 and II-2 depict two signal arrays of very different quality, detected from very different muscles. They provide two extreme examples of possible EMG signals.

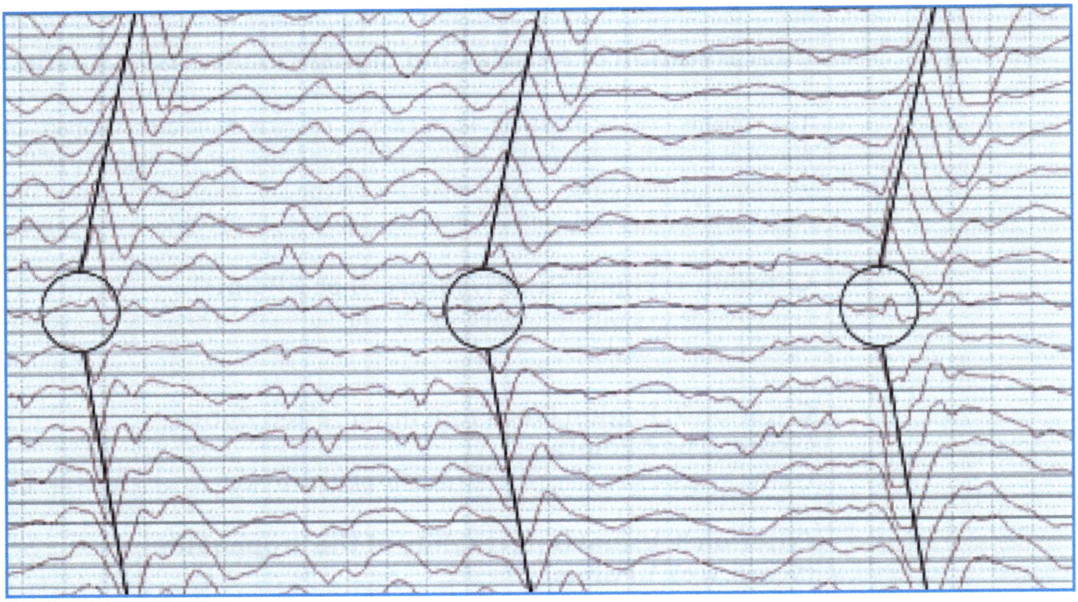

**Fig. II.1** Surface EMG signals detected from the short head of the biceps brachii during an isometric contraction, as detected using a linear electrode array (5 ms/div). In this case, signals were detectable without noise (criterion 1, score 2). The *black circles* indicate a clearly visible innervation zone (IZ) and the propagation of motor unit action potentials is detectable from several channels along the *black lines* (criterion 4, score 1). Given an inter-electrode distance of 5 mm, two wide areas (5 mm × 7 channels = 35 mm, proximally and distally with respect to the IZ) are available for bipolar electrode placement (criterion 2, score 2). The slope of the black lines is a rough estimate of muscle-fiber conduction velocity within the physiological range (4–5 m/s) (criterion 3, score 1)

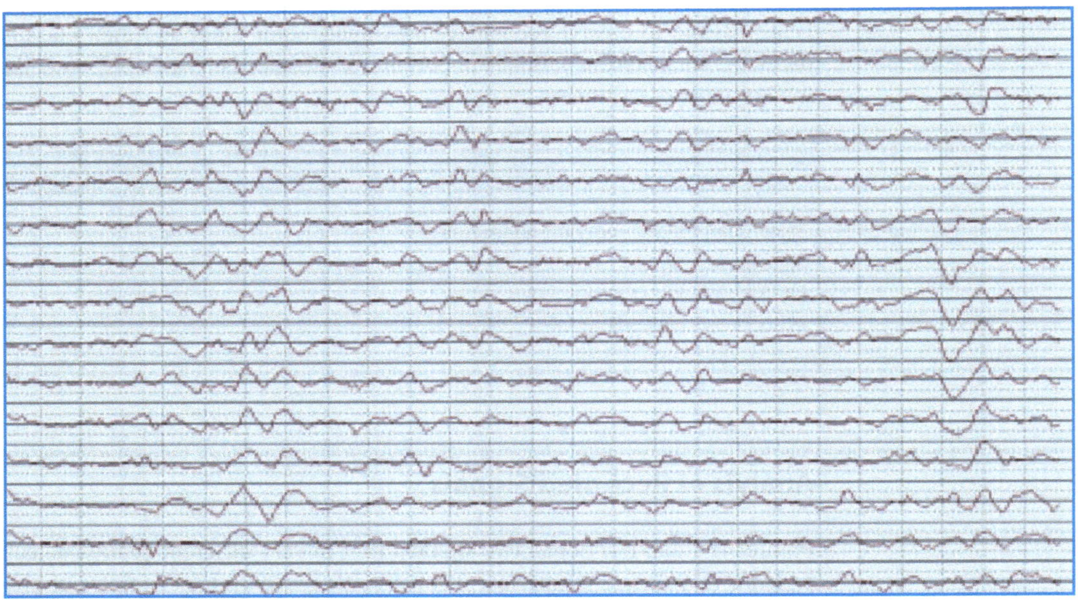

**Fig. II.2** Surface EMG signals from the soleus muscle, detected during an isometric contraction using a linear electrode array (5 ms/div). In this case, good signals were not detectable due to noise, end-of-fiber, or cross-talk effects (criterion 1, score 0). Motor-unit action potentials and their propagation were not identifiable (criterion 3 and 4, score 0). No IZ is visible. An electrode pair can be placed in any location over the region covered by the array (criterion 2, score2)

## Interpretation of Tables in This Atlas

In the following, a sample table is provided, with a detailed description of the information that can be extracted.

- **Anatomical landmark frames (ALF)**: A line from the center of the inferior point of the mastoid process to the center of the sternal notch.
- **Experimental set up**: The subject was seated with his or her head rigidly fixed in a device for the measurement of multi-directional neck force, the back supported, knees and hips in 90° flexion, the torso firmly strapped to the seat back, and the hands resting comfortably in the lap. He or she then performed an isometric neck flexion. (2)
- **Optimal electrode site**: Between 0% and 48% of the ALF.
- **Notes**: In all 40 subjects, the propagation of motor unit action potentials was clearly seen.

| Subjects investigated | IZs detected (3) |
|---|---|
| 20 Males | 20 |
| 20 Females | 20 |

| Results (4) | |
|---|---|
| Min | 48% |
| 1st quartile | 59% |
| Median | 64% |
| 3rd quartile | 71% |
| Max | 81% |

| Quality analysis (5) | | |
|---|---|---|
| **Items** | **Values** | **Score** |
| **1** Signal quality | 0 or 2 | 2 |
| **2** Area without IZ | 0 or 2 | 2 |
| **3** Physiological signal propagation | 0 or 1 | 1 |
| **4** Motor units identification | 0 or 1 | 1 |
| Total | | 6 |

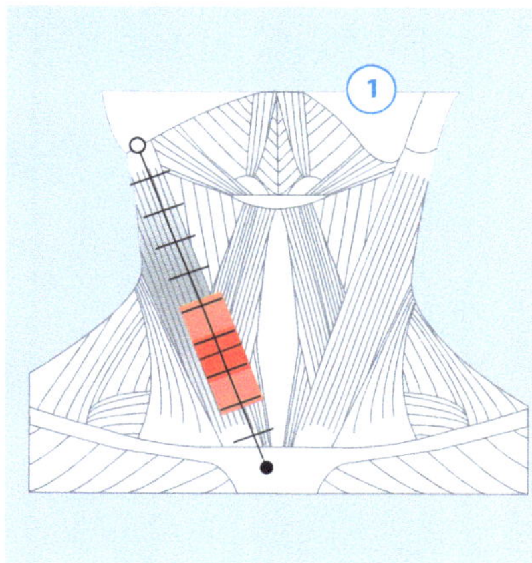


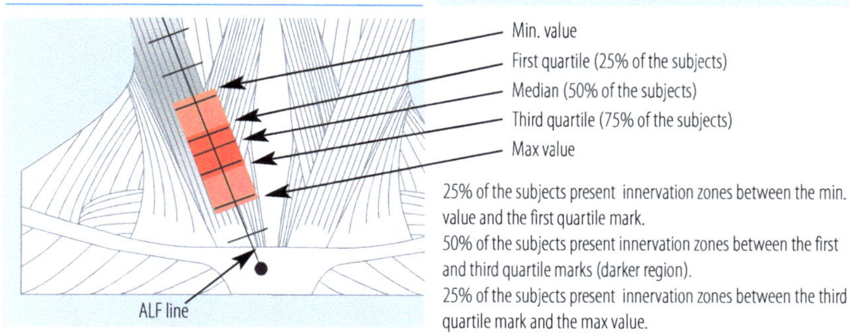


In each anatomical illustration the investigated muscle is colored in dark gray (*1*) and the line indicating the anatomical landmark frame (ALF) is applied according to the starting point (*empty circle*) and the ending point (*filled circle*). A detailed description is also reported in (*2*), together with the positioning of the subject for measurements of isometric muscle contraction. In (*3*), the numbers of studied (male and female) subjects are reported along with the number of detected IZs. In (*4*), numerical values of the "box and whiskers" plot are reported in order to allow the reader to assess the optimal electrode site (last row in 2). Finally, a qualitative multi-criteria score (see pag 83 for the description) is shown in (*5*). It provides the reader with an immediate tool for comparing the different signals.

# Trunk

# Sternocleidomastoid

- **Anatomical landmark frames (ALF)**: A line from the center of the inferior point of the mastoid process to the center of the sternal notch.
- **Experimental set up**: The subject was seated with his or her head rigidly fixed in a device for the measurement of multi-directional neck force, the back supported, knees and hips in 90° flexion, the torso firmly strapped to the seat back, and the hands resting comfortably in the lap. He or she then performed an isometric neck flexion.
- **Optimal electrode site**: Between 0% and 48% of the ALF.
- **Notes**: In all 40 subjects, the propagation of motor unit action potentials was clearly seen.

| Subjects investigated | IZs detected |
|---|---|
| 20 Males | 20 |
| 20 Females | 20 |

| Results | |
|---|---|
| Min | 48% |
| 1st quartile | 59% |
| Median | 64% |
| 3rd quartile | 71% |
| Max | 81% |

| Quality analysis | | |
|---|---|---|
| Items | Values | Score |
| **1** Signal quality | 0 or 2 | 2 |
| **2** Area without IZ | 0 or 2 | 2 |
| **3** Physiological signal propagation | 0 or 1 | 1 |
| **4** Motor units identification | 0 or 1 | 1 |
| Total | | 6 |

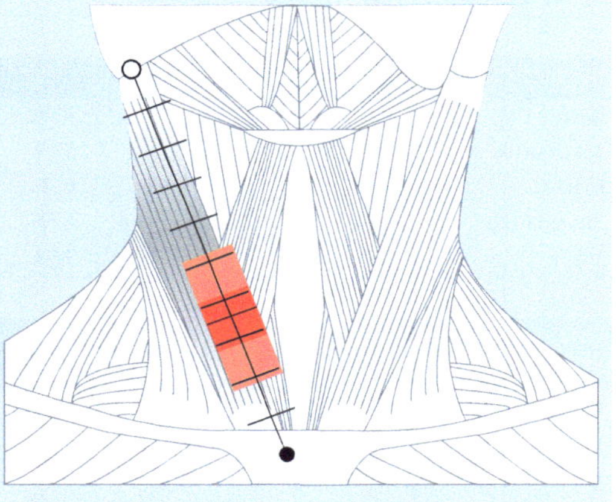

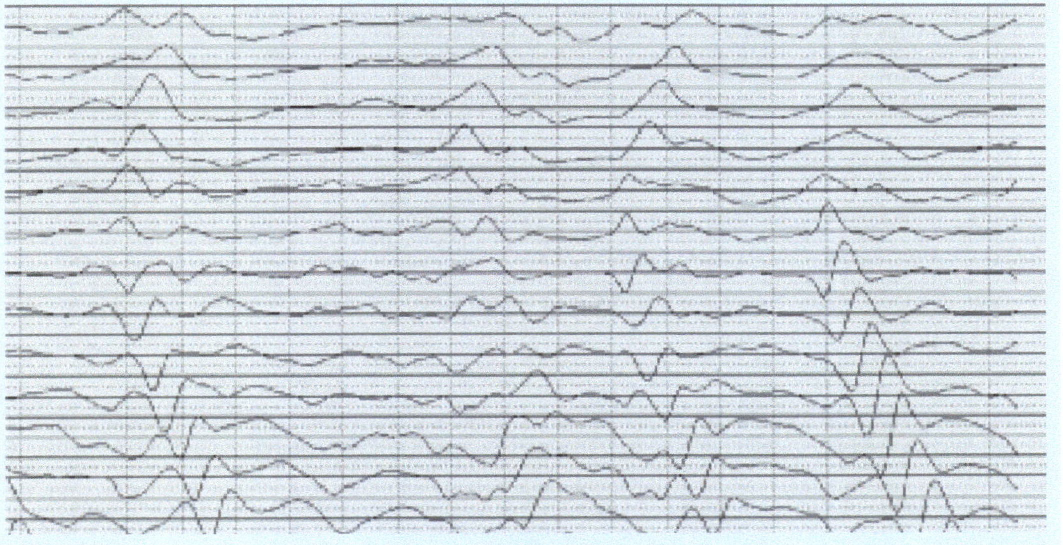

5 ms/division

## Pectoralis Major

- **Anatomical landmark frames (ALF)**: A line between the acromial angle and the xiphoid process of the sternum.
- **Experimental set up**: The subject was standing with one arm abducted at about 30°. He or she then performed an isometric contraction during an adduction of the arm.
- **Optimal electrode site**: On the muscle belly, between 0% and 45% or between 76% and 100% of the ALF. The probe was laterally inclined with respect to the ALF.
- **Notes**: In all 20 male subjects, but in none of the 20 female subjects, the propagation of motor unit action potentials was clearly seen.

| Subjects investigated | IZs detected |
|---|---|
| 20 Males | 20 |
| 20 Females | 0 |

| Results | |
|---|---|
| Min | 45% |
| 1st quartile | 57% |
| Median | 62% |
| 3rd quartile | 67% |
| Max | 76% |

| Quality analysis | | | |
|---|---|---|---|
| | Items | Values | Score |
| **1** | Signal quality | 0 or 2 | 2 |
| **2** | Area without IZ | 0 or 2 | 2 |
| **3** | Physiological signal propagation | 0 or 1 | 0 |
| **4** | Motor units identification | 0 or 1 | 0 |
| | Total | | 4 |

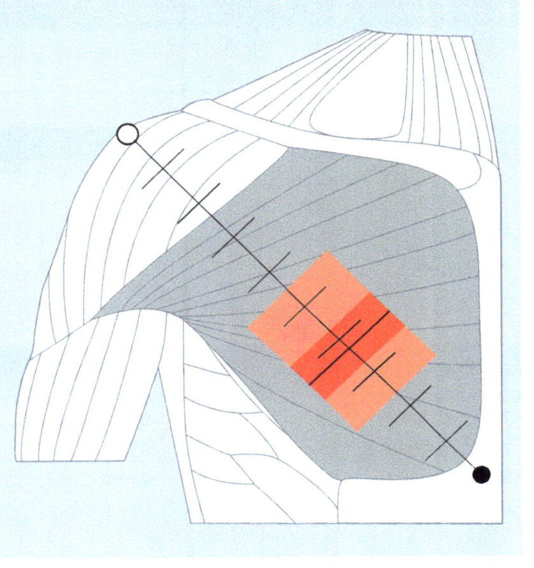

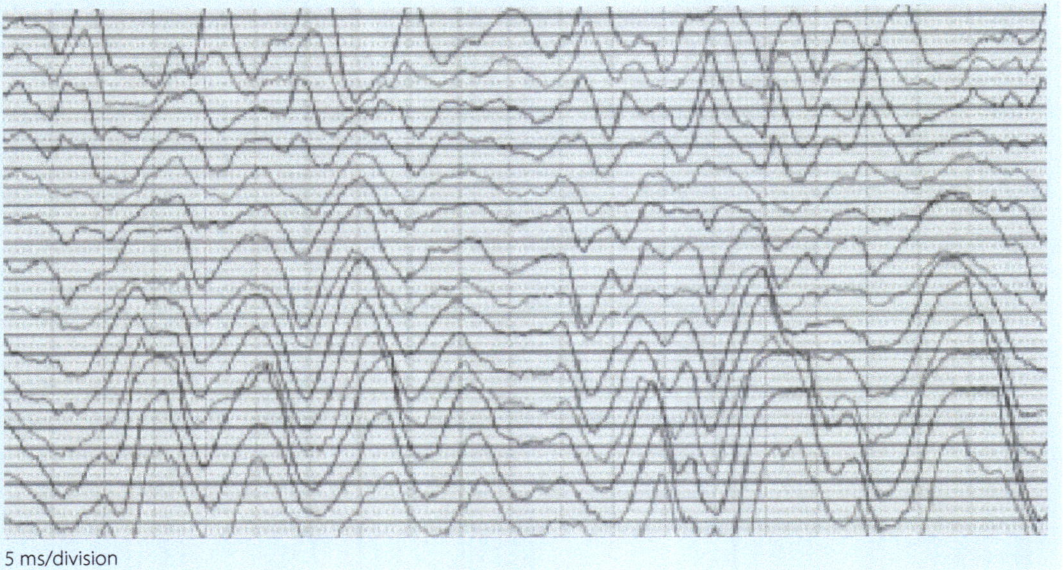

5 ms/division

## Serratus Anterior

- **Anatomical landmark frames (ALF)**: An effective ALF could not be drawn. The probes were positioned, according to the direction of the fibers, on the available muscle belly between the fifth and seventh ribs.
- **Experimental set up**: The subject was placed in the supine position with one arm extended at 90°. He or she then performed an isometric contraction during an upward thrust of the fist.
- **Optimal electrode site**: Anywhere on the available muscle belly.
- **Notes**: All 40 subjects showed clear signal propagation, but no IZs were detected as they were located somewhere under the scapula.

| Subjects investigated | IZs detected |
|---|---|
| 20 Males | 0 |
| 20 Females | 0 |

**Results: None**

| Quality analysis | | | |
|---|---|---|---|
| | Items | Values | Score |
| **1** | Signal quality | 0 or 2 | 2 |
| **2** | Area without IZ | 0 or 2 | 2 |
| **3** | Physiological signal propagation | 0 or 1 | 1 |
| **4** | Motor units identification | 0 or 1 | 1 |
| | Total | | 6 |

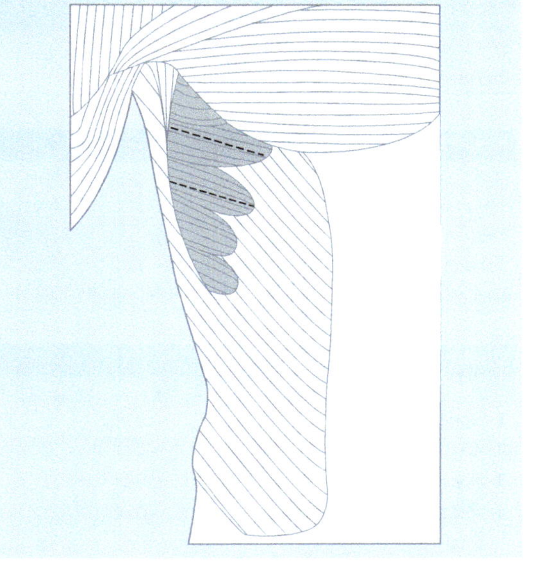

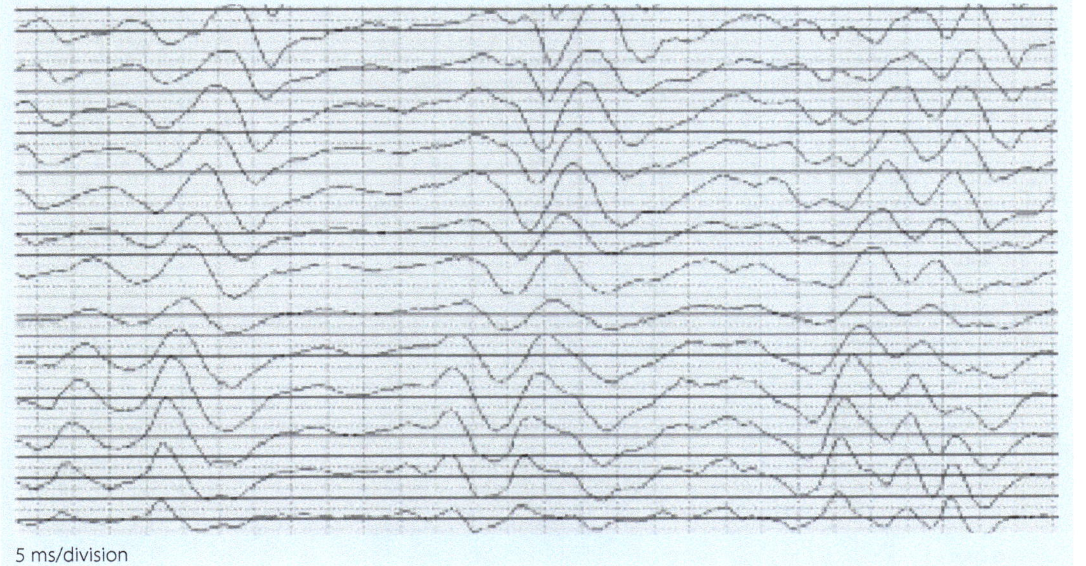

5 ms/division

# Rectus Abdominis: Superior (I)

- **Anatomical landmark frames (ALF)**: A line on the right portion of the muscle belly parallel to the linea alba. The line starts at the level of the xiphoid process and ends at the level of the superior anterior iliac spine.
- **Experimental set up**: The subject was placed in the supine position. He or she then performed an isometric contraction during trunk flexion.
- **Optimal electrode site**: Between 0% and 13% of the ALF.
- **Notes**: Since the rectus abdominis is a multi-segmented muscle, three IZs were detected based on the ALF. The rectus abdominis is composed of five muscle bellies divided by tendinous intersections; the muscle bellies vary in size and the tendinous intersections are not always palpable. Therefore, it was not possible to establish an optimal electrode site.

| Subjects investigated | IZs detected |
|---|---|
| 20 Males | 20 |
| 20 Females | 20 |

| Results | |
|---|---|
| Min | 13% |
| 1st quartile | 16% |
| Median | 21% |
| 3rd quartile | 25% |
| Max | 29% |

| Quality analysis | | |
|---|---|---|
| **Items** | **Values** | **Score** |
| **1** Signal quality | 0 or 2 | 2 |
| **2** Area without IZ | 0 or 2 | 2 |
| **3** Physiological signal propagation | 0 or 1 | 1 |
| **4** Motor units identification | 0 or 1 | 1 |
| Total | | 6 |

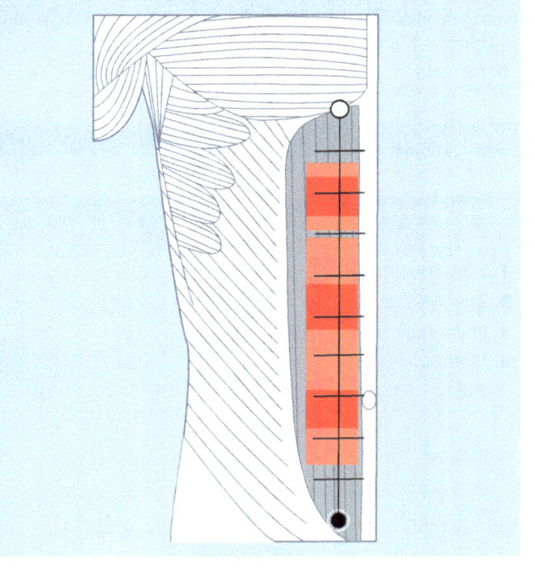

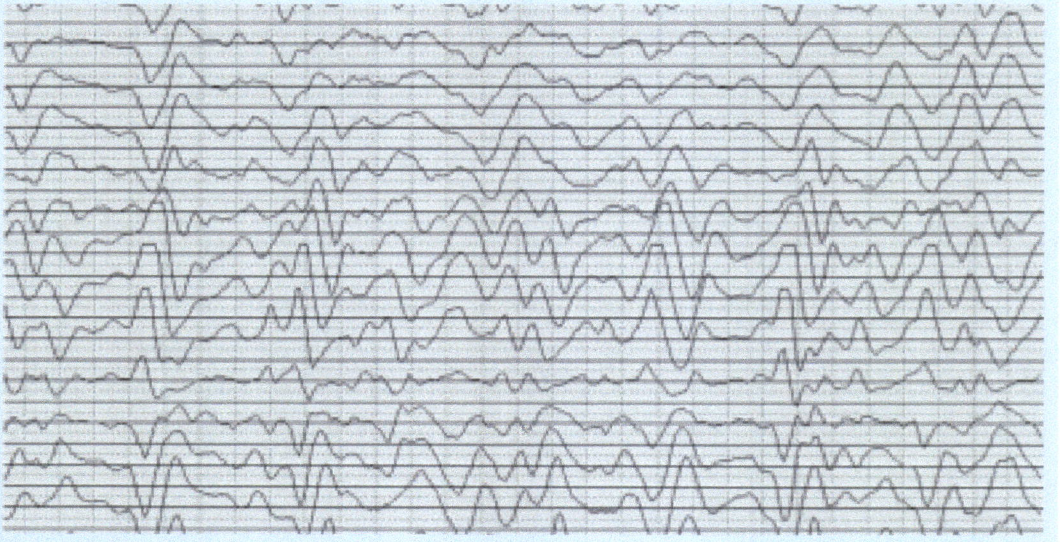

5 ms/division

# Rectus Abdominis: Middle (II)

- **Anatomical landmark frames (ALF)**: A line on the right portion of the muscle belly parallel to the linea alba. The line starts at the level of the xiphoid process and ends at the level of the superior anterior iliac spine.
- **Experimental set up**: The subject was placed in the supine position. He or she then performed an isometric contraction during trunk flexion.
- **Optimal electrode site**: Not applicable.
- **Notes**: Since the rectus abdominis is a multi-segmented muscle, three IZs were detected based on the ALF. The rectus abdominis is composed of five muscle bellies divided by tendinous intersections. The muscle bellies vary in size and the tendinous intersections are not always palpable. Therefore, it was not possible to establish an optimal electrode site.

| Subjects investigated | IZs detected |
|---|---|
| 20 Males | 20 |
| 20 Females | 20 |

| Results | |
|---|---|
| Min | 31% |
| 1st quartile | 43% |
| Median | 48% |
| 3rd quartile | 53% |
| Max | 63% |

| Quality analysis | | | |
|---|---|---|---|
| | Items | Values | Score |
| 1 | Signal quality | 0 or 2 | 2 |
| 2 | Area without IZ | 0 or 2 | 0 |
| 3 | Physiological signal propagation | 0 or 1 | 1 |
| 4 | Motor units identification | 0 or 1 | 1 |
| | Total | | 4 |

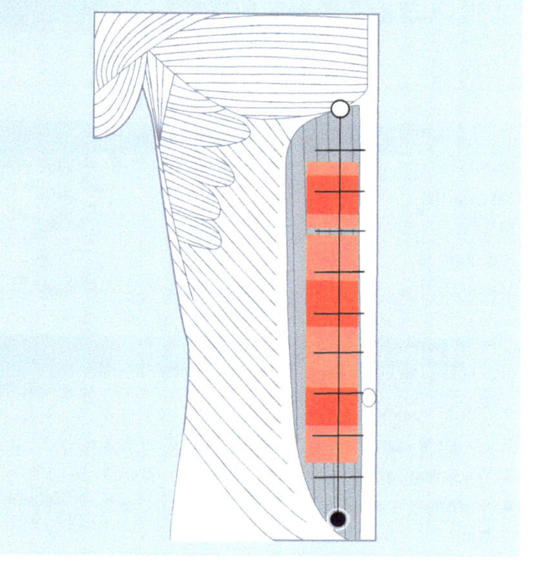

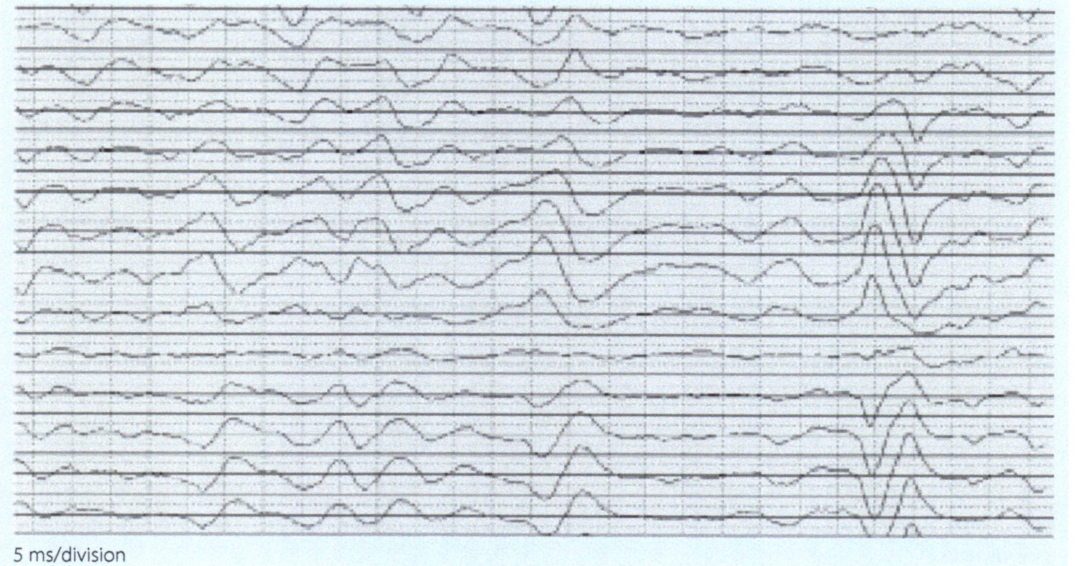

5 ms/division

# Rectus Abdominis: Inferior (III)

- **Anatomical landmark frames (ALF)**: A line on the right portion of the muscle belly parallel to the linea alba. The line starts at the level of the xiphoid process and ends at the level of the superior anterior iliac spine.
- **Experimental set up**: The subject was placed in the supine position. He or she then performed an isometric contraction during trunk flexion.
- **Optimal electrode site**: Between 86% and 100% of the ALF.
- **Notes**: Since the rectus abdominis is a multi-segmented muscle, three IZs were detected based on the ALF. The rectus abdominis is composed of five muscle bellies divided by tendinous intersections; the muscle bellies vary in size and the tendinous intersections are not always palpable. Therefore, it was not possible to establish an optimal electrode site.

| Subjects investigated | IZs detected |
|---|---|
| 20 Males | 20 |
| 20 Females | 20 |

| Results | |
|---|---|
| Min | 54% |
| 1st quartile | 68% |
| Median | 72% |
| 3rd quartile | 77% |
| Max | 86% |

| Quality analysis | | | |
|---|---|---|---|
| | Items | Values | Score |
| 1 | Signal quality | 0 or 2 | 2 |
| 2 | Area without IZ | 0 or 2 | 2 |
| 3 | Physiological signal propagation | 0 or 1 | 1 |
| 4 | Motor units identification | 0 or 1 | 1 |
| | Total | | 6 |

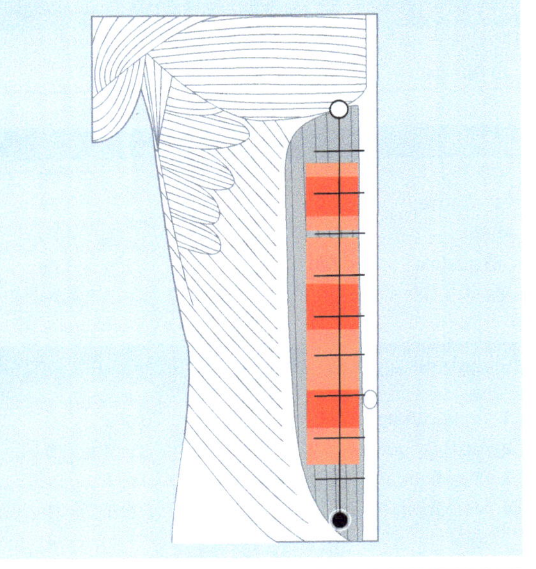

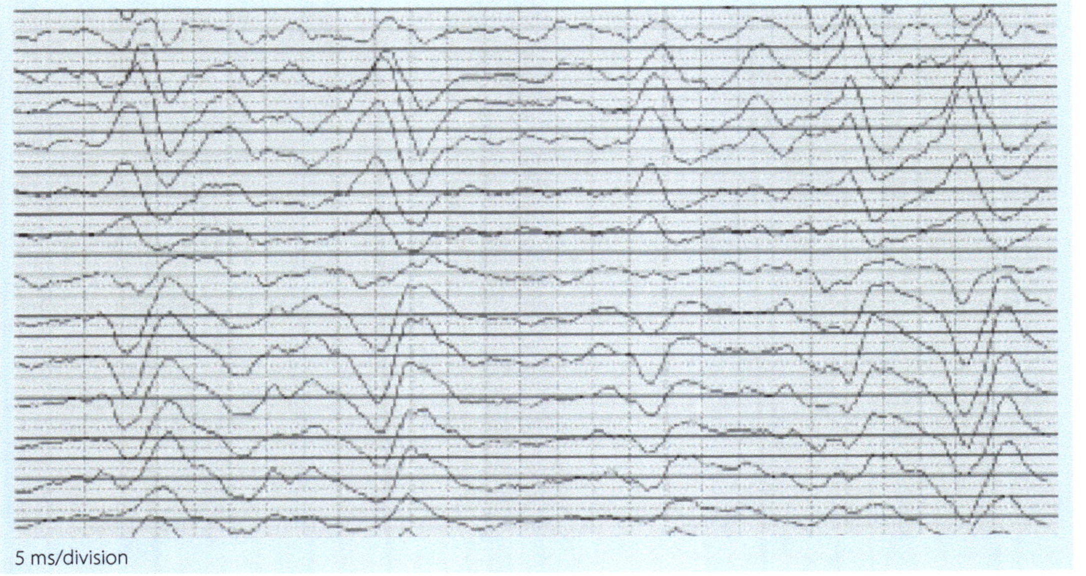

5 ms/division

# Upper Trapezius

- **Anatomical landmark frames (ALF)**: A line from the distal portion of the clavicle to the spinal process of the sixth cervical vertebrae.
- **Experimental set up**: The subject was seated with his or her arm abducted at 90°. An isometric contraction was then performed during elevation of the shoulders.
- **Optimal electrode site**: Between 0% and 44% or between 72% and 100% of the ALF.

| Subjects investigated | IZs detected |
|---|---|
| 20 Males | 20 |
| 20 Females | 20 |

| Results | |
|---|---|
| Min | 44% |
| 1st quartile | 55% |
| Median | 58% |
| 3rd quartile | 59% |
| Max | 72% |

| Quality analysis | | |
|---|---|---|
| **Items** | **Values** | **Score** |
| **1** Signal quality | 0 or 2 | 2 |
| **2** Area without IZ | 0 or 2 | 2 |
| **3** Physiological signal propagation | 0 or 1 | 1 |
| **4** Motor units identification | 0 or 1 | 1 |
| Total | | 6 |

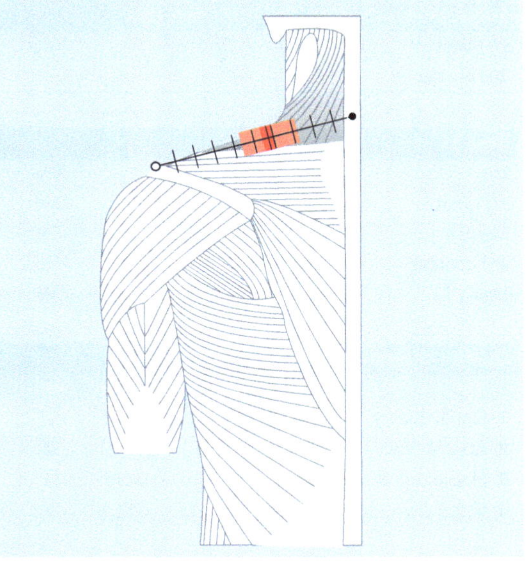

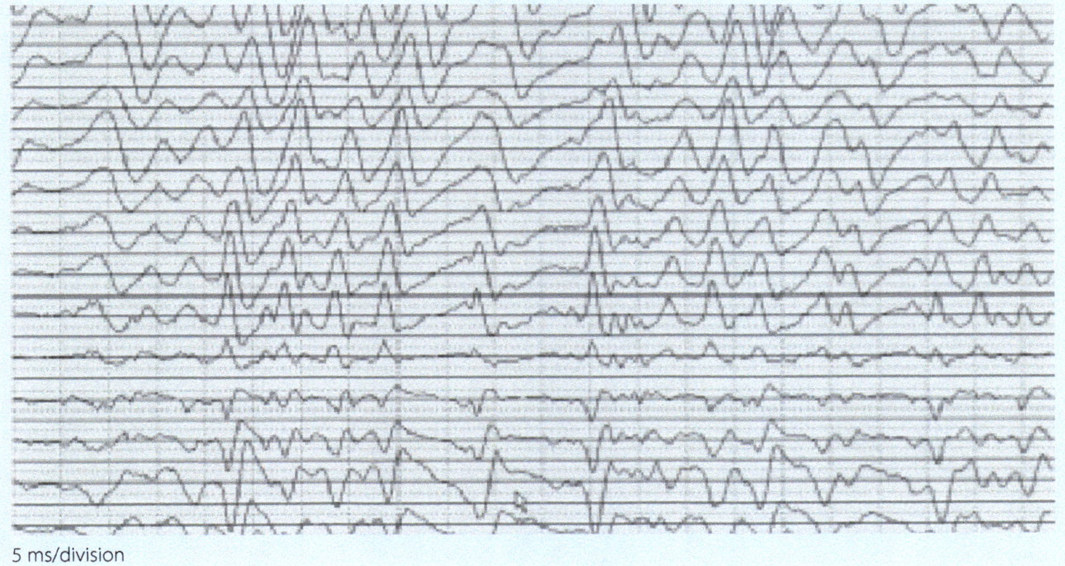

5 ms/division

# Middle Trapezius

- **Anatomical landmark frames (ALF)**: A line between the spinous process of the seventh cervical vertebrae and the acromial angle.
- **Experimental set up**: The subject was seated on a chair grasping a fixed handles. He or she then performed an isometric contraction during elevation of the shoulders.
- **Optimal electrode site**: Between 0% and 35% or between 70% and 100% of the ALF.
- **Notes**: In all 40 subjects, the propagation of motor unit action potentials was clearly seen.

| Subjects investigated | IZs detected |
|---|---|
| 20 Males | 20 |
| 20 Females | 20 |

| Results | |
|---|---|
| Min | 35% |
| 1st quartile | 43% |
| Median | 46% |
| 3rd quartile | 48% |
| Max | 70% |

| Quality analysis | | |
|---|---|---|
| Items | Values | Score |
| **1** Signal quality | 0 or 2 | 2 |
| **2** Area without IZ | 0 or 2 | 2 |
| **3** Physiological signal propagation | 0 or 1 | 1 |
| **4** Motor units identification | 0 or 1 | 1 |
| Total | | 6 |

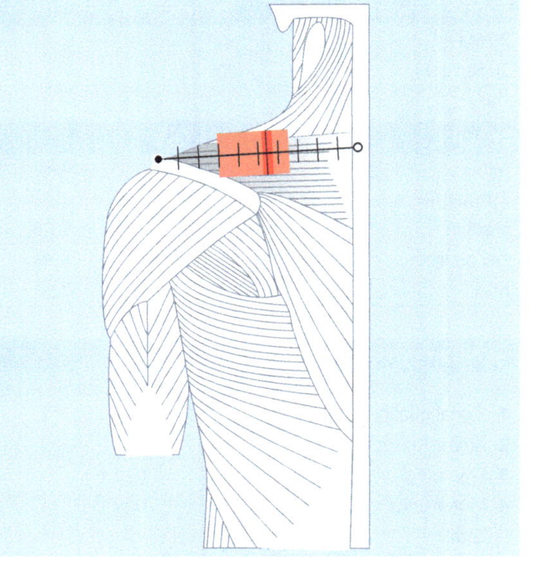

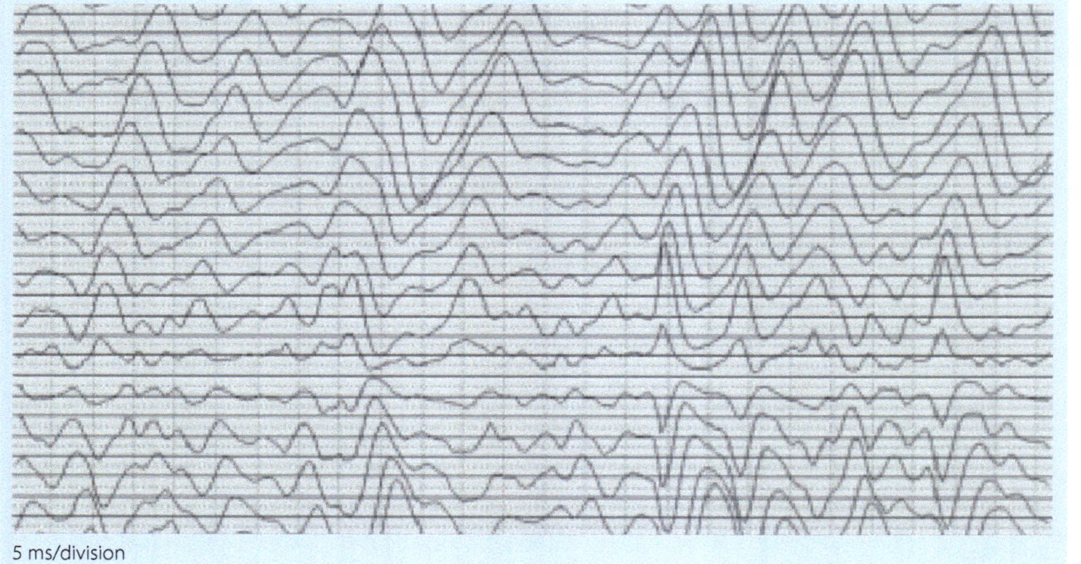

5 ms/division

## Lower Trapezius

- **Anatomical landmark frames (ALF)**: A line between the scapular spine and the spinous process of the twelfth thoracic vertebrae.
- **Experimental set up**: The subject lay on his or her left side with the right arm flexed at 90°. An isometric contraction was then performed with horizontal abduction.
- **Optimal electrode site**: Between 0% and 22% or between 52% and 100% of the ALF.

| Subjects investigated | IZs detected |
|---|---|
| 20 Males | 20 |
| 20 Females | 20 |

| Results | |
|---|---|
| Min | 22% |
| 1st quartile | 26% |
| Median | 33% |
| 3rd quartile | 35% |
| Max | 52% |

| Quality analysis | | | |
|---|---|---|---|
| | Items | Values | Score |
| 1 | Signal quality | 0 or 2 | 2 |
| 2 | Area without IZ | 0 or 2 | 2 |
| 3 | Physiological signal propagation | 0 or 1 | 1 |
| 4 | Motor units identification | 0 or 1 | 1 |
| | Total | | 6 |

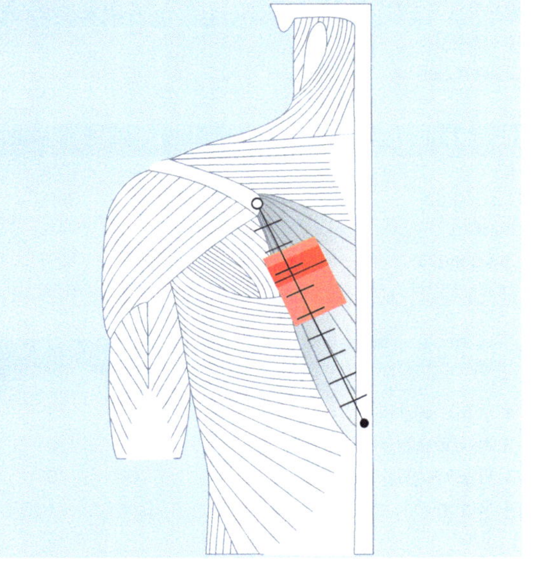

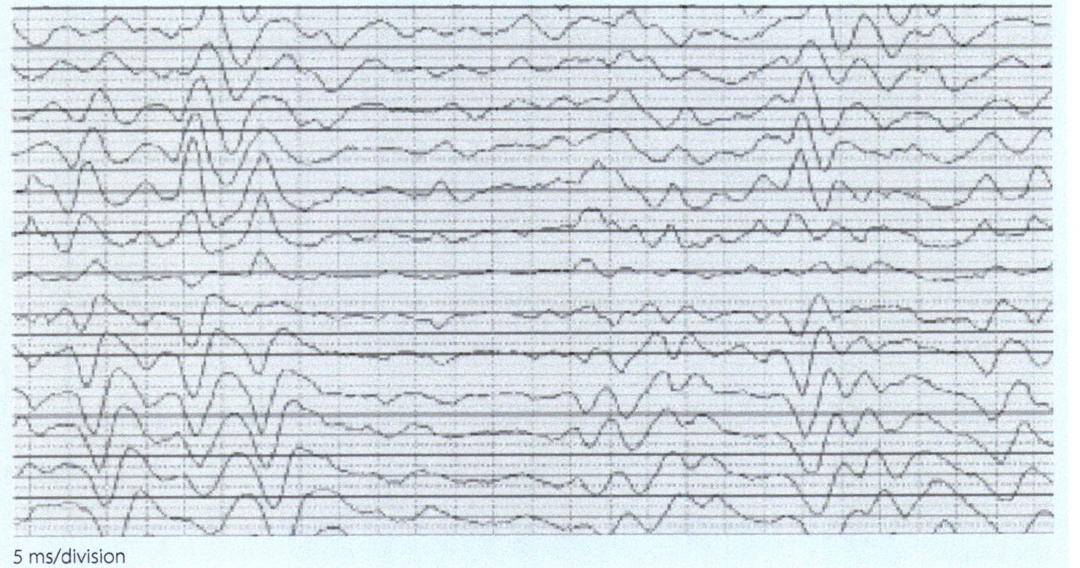

5 ms/division

# Rhomboid Major

- **Anatomical landmark frames (ALF)**: A line between the spinous of the third thoracic vertebrae and the medial border of the scapula. The line was drawn at an angle of 45° to the sagittal plane.
- **Experimental set up**: The subject was seated on a chair with his or her left arm at 90° of abduction and the forearm flexed at 90°. An isometric contraction was then performed during a horizontal extension.
- **Optimal electrode site**: Between 0% and 25% or between 66% and 100% of the ALF.
- **Notes**: In the 20 male subjects, the propagation of motor unit action potentials was clearly seen. In three of the 20 females, determination of the IZ was not possible due to low-quality signals.

| Subjects investigated | IZs detected |
|---|---|
| 20 Males | 20 |
| 20 Females | 20 |

| Results | |
|---|---|
| Min | 25% |
| 1st quartile | 38% |
| Median | 44% |
| 3rd quartile | 50% |
| Max | 63% |

| Quality analysis | | | |
|---|---|---|---|
| | Items | Values | Score |
| **1** | Signal quality | 0 or 2 | 2 |
| **2** | Area without IZ | 0 or 2 | 2 |
| **3** | Physiological signal propagation | 0 or 1 | 0 |
| **4** | Motor units identification | 0 or 1 | 1 |
| | Total | | 5 |

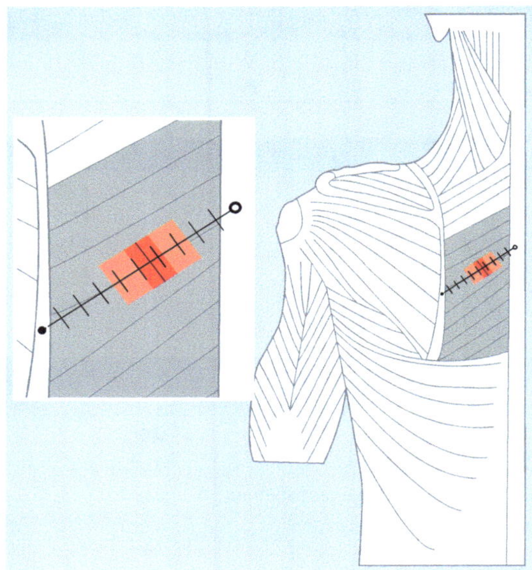

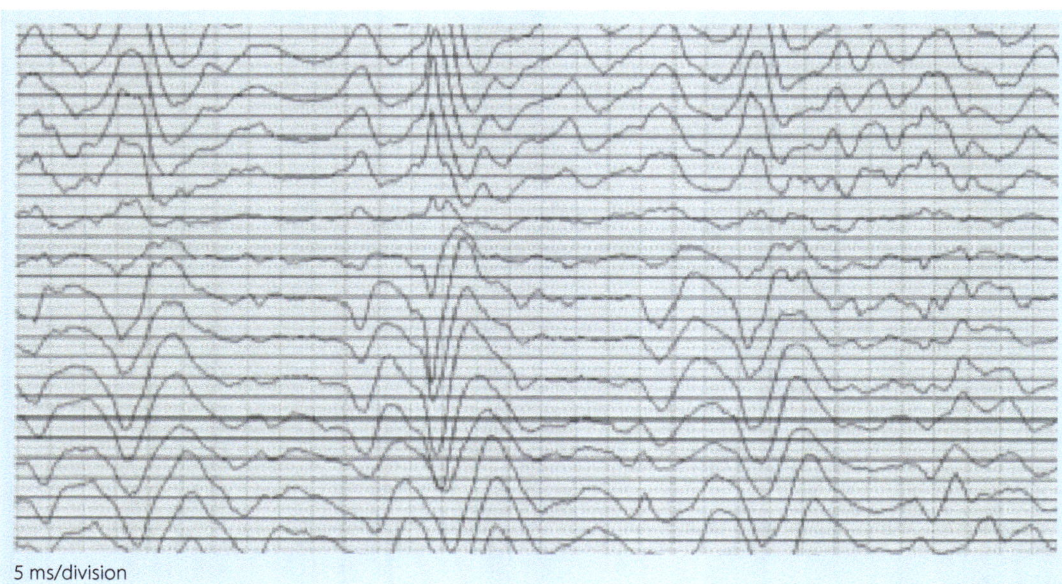

## Rhomboid Minor

- **Anatomical landmark frames (ALF)**: A line between the spinous process of the seventh cervical vertebrae and the medial border of the scapula. The line was drawn at an angle of 45° to the sagittal plane.
- **Experimental set up**: The subject was seated on a chair with his or her left arm at 90° of abduction and the forearm flexed at 90°. An isometric contraction was then performed during a horizontal extension.
- **Optimal electrode site**: Between 0% and 36% of the ALF.
- **Notes**: In the 20 male subjects, the propagation of motor unit action potentials was clearly seen. In three of the 20 females, IZ determination was not possible due to low-quality signals.

| Subjects investigated | IZs detected |
|---|---|
| 20 Males | 20 |
| 20 Females | 20 |

| Results | |
|---|---|
| Min | 36% |
| 1st quartile | 55% |
| Median | 63% |
| 3rd quartile | 72% |
| Max | 94% |

| Quality analysis | | |
|---|---|---|
| **Items** | **Values** | **Score** |
| **1** Signal quality | 0 or 2 | 2 |
| **2** Area without IZ | 0 or 2 | 2 |
| **3** Physiological signal propagation | 0 or 1 | 1 |
| **4** Motor units identification | 0 or 1 | 1 |
| Total | | 6 |

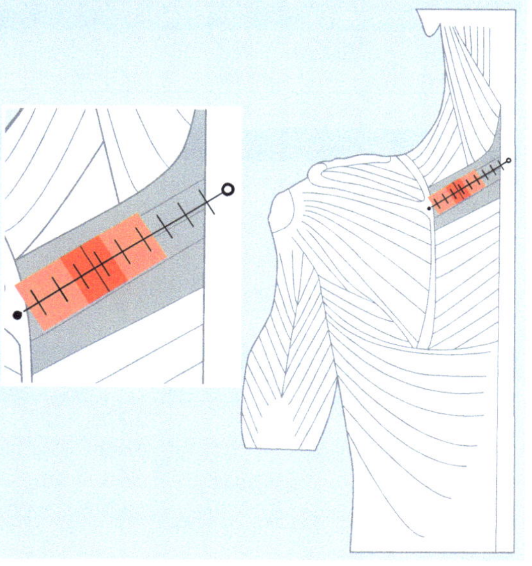

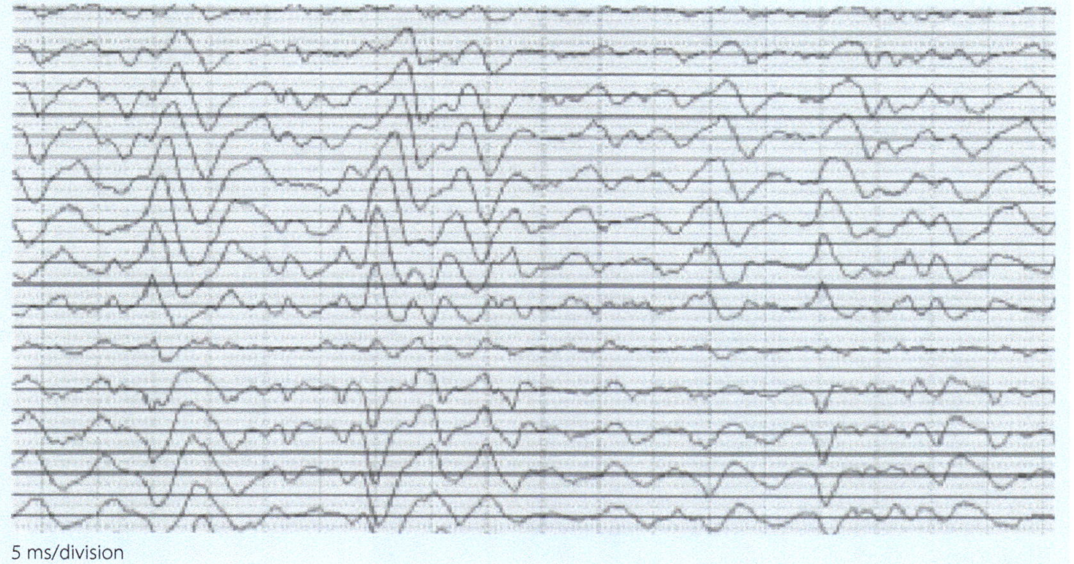

5 ms/division

# Infraspinatus

- **Anatomical landmark frames (ALF)**: A line from the midpoint of the scapular medial border to the greater tubercle.
- **Experimental set up**: The subject was seated with his or her forearm flexed at 90°. An isometric contraction against resistance was performed during an external rotation.
- **Optimal electrode site**: Between 40% and 100% of the ALF.

| Subjects investigated | IZs detected |
|---|---|
| 20 Males | 20 |
| 20 Females | 20 |

| Results | |
|---|---|
| Min | 8% |
| 1st quartile | 17% |
| Median | 23% |
| 3rd quartile | 27% |
| Max | 40% |

| Quality analysis | | | |
|---|---|---|---|
| | Items | Values | Score |
| 1 | Signal quality | 0 or 2 | 2 |
| 2 | Area without IZ | 0 or 2 | 2 |
| 3 | Physiological signal propagation | 0 or 1 | 0 |
| 4 | Motor units identification | 0 or 1 | 1 |
| | Total | | 5 |

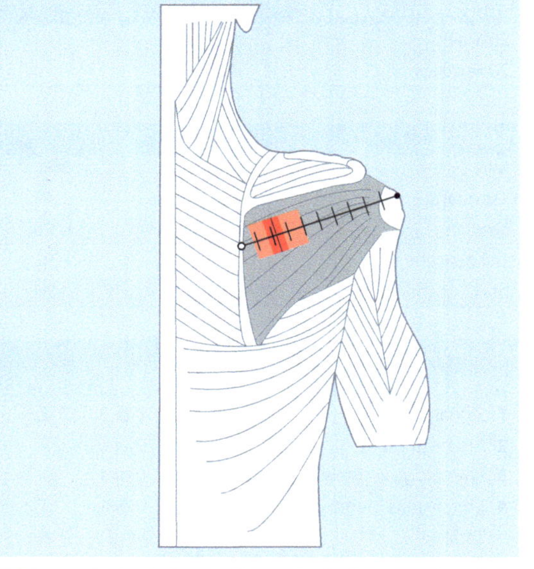

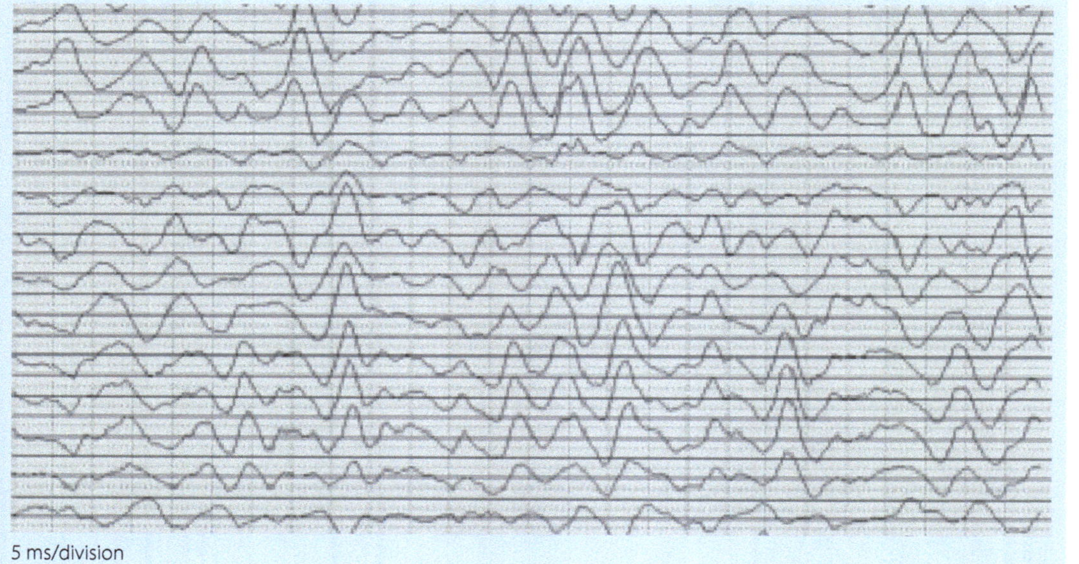

5 ms/division

# Latissimus Dorsi

- **Anatomical landmark frames (ALF)**: A line from the posterior superior iliac spine to the midpoint of a line between the greater tubercle and the spinal process of the fifth lumbar vertebrae.
- **Experimental set up**: The subject was seated with his or her forearm flexed at 90°. An isometric contraction against resistance was performed during an extension of the arm associated with a depression of the shoulders.
- **Optimal electrode site**: Between 0% and 16% or between 55% and 100% of the ALF.
- **Notes**: In case of a distal positioning of the electrode, the ALF will partially overlap the thoracolumbar fascia.

| Subjects investigated | IZs detected |
|---|---|
| 20 Males | 20 |
| 20 Females | 20 |

| Results | |
|---|---|
| Min | 16% |
| 1st quartile | 24% |
| Median | 31% |
| 3rd quartile | 36% |
| Max | 55% |

| Quality analysis | | | |
|---|---|---|---|
| | Items | Values | Score |
| **1** | Signal quality | 0 or 2 | 2 |
| **2** | Area without IZ | 0 or 2 | 2 |
| **3** | Physiological signal propagation | 0 or 1 | 0 |
| **4** | Motor units identification | 0 or 1 | 1 |
| | Total | | 5 |

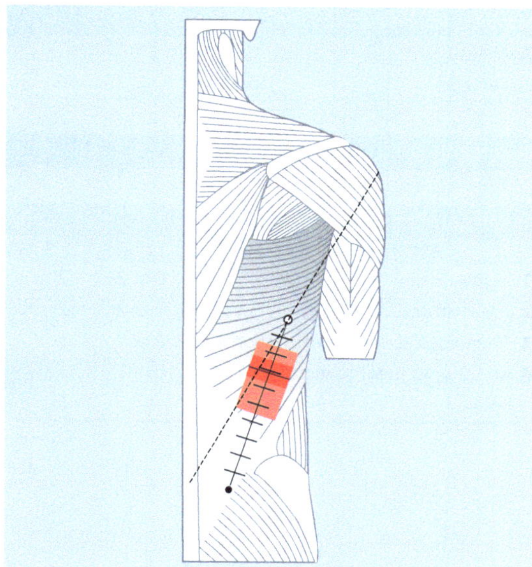

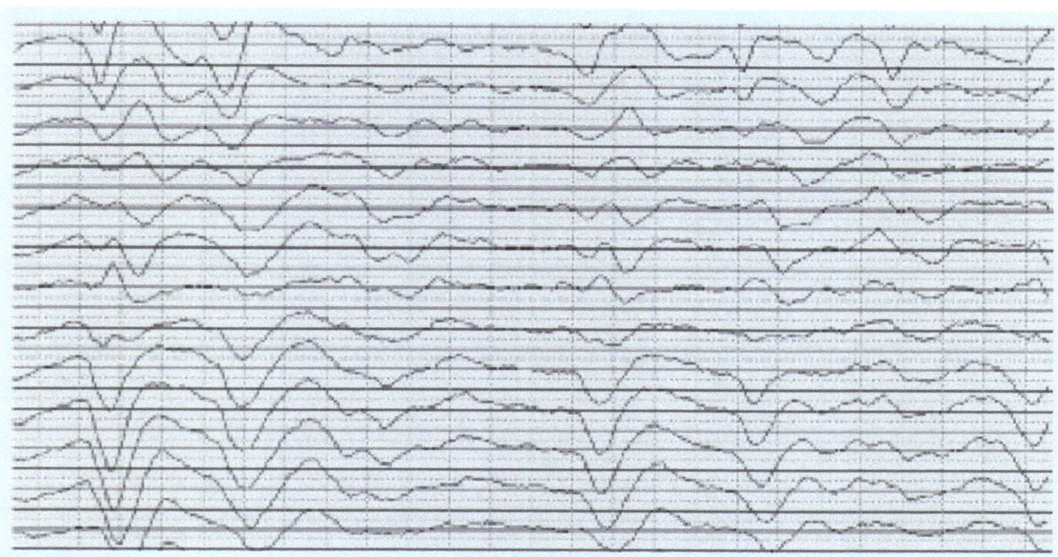

5 ms/division

# Erector Spinae

- **Anatomical landmark frames (ALF)**: A line between the spinal processes of the fifth lumbar vertebrae and the twelfth thoracic vertebrae, 1 cm laterally on the muscle belly.
- **Experimental set up**: The subject was placed in the prone position. He or she then performed an isometric contraction during trunk extension.
- **Optimal electrode site**: A unique optimal electrode site could not be defined since electrode can be optimally placed throughout the ALF and since no IZs were detected.

| Subjects investigated | IZs detected |
|---|---|
| 20 Males | 0 |
| 20 Females | 0 |

**Results: None**

| Quality analysis | | |
|---|---|---|
| **Items** | **Values** | **Score** |
| **1** Signal quality | 0 or 2 | 2 |
| **2** Area without IZ | 0 or 2 | 2 |
| **3** Physiological signal propagation | 0 or 1 | 1 |
| **4** Motor units identification | 0 or 1 | 1 |
| Total | | 6 |

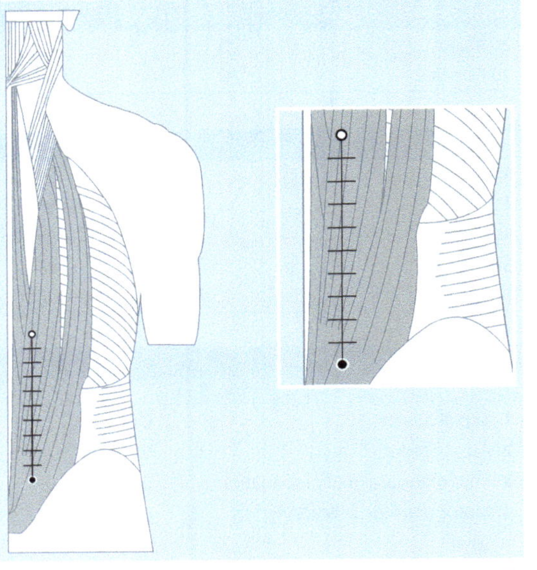

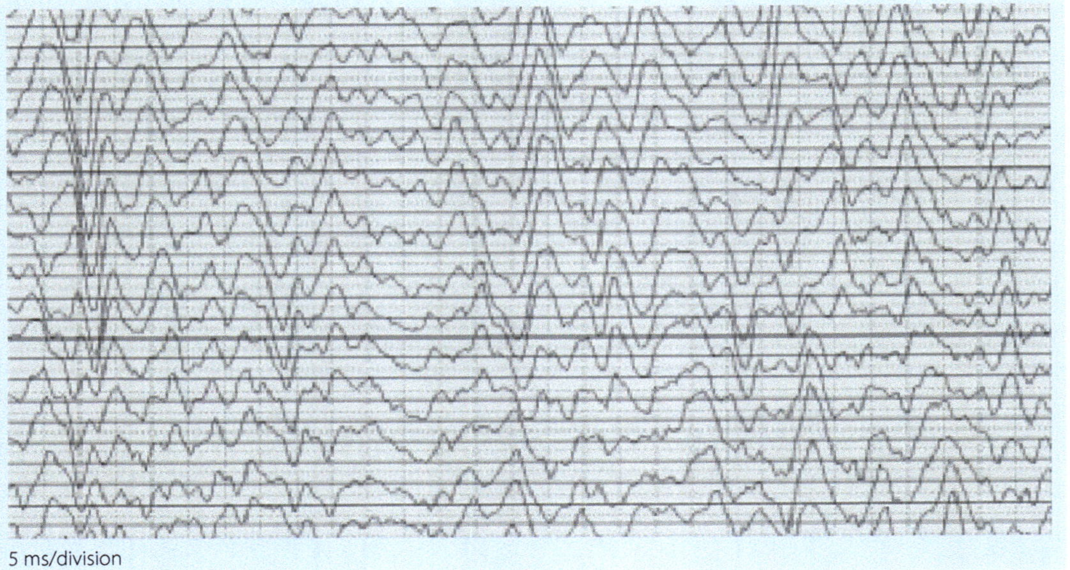

5 ms/division

# Upper Limb

# Posterior Deltoid

- **Anatomical landmark frames (ALF)**: The probe was placed perpendicular to the line extending from the acromion to the center of the glenoid cavity.
- **Experimental set up**: The subject was seated with his or her arm abducted at 90° and the elbow flexed. An isometric contraction was then performed during retropulsion of the arm against a resistance applied at elbow level.
- **Optimal electrode site**: Perpendicular to the ALF at about 47% of its length, at a medial or lateral distance along the muscle belly > 2 cm.
- **Notes**: In 39 of the 40 subjects, the propagation of motor unit action potentials was clearly seen.

| Subjects investigated | IZs detected |
|---|---|
| 20 Males | 20 |
| 20 Females | 19 |

| Results | |
|---|---|
| Min | 32% |
| 1st quartile | 42% |
| Median | 47% |
| 3rd quartile | 50% |
| Max | 62% |

| Quality analysis | | |
|---|---|---|
| **Items** | **Values** | **Score** |
| **1** Signal quality | 0 or 2 | 2 |
| **2** Area without IZ | 0 or 2 | 2 |
| **3** Physiological signal propagation | 0 or 1 | 1 |
| **4** Motor units identification | 0 or 1 | 1 |
| Total | | 6 |

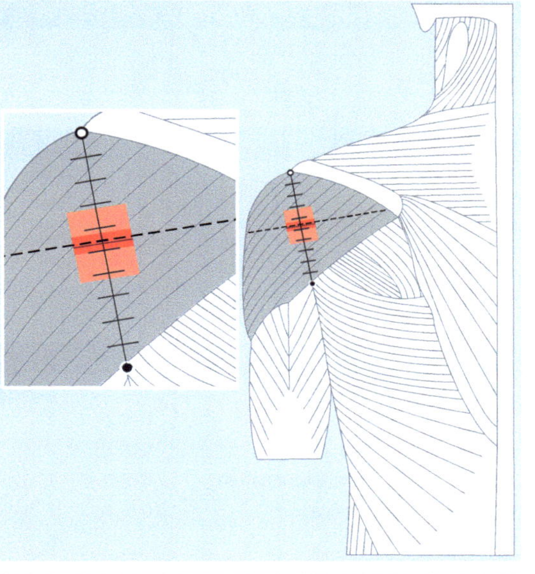

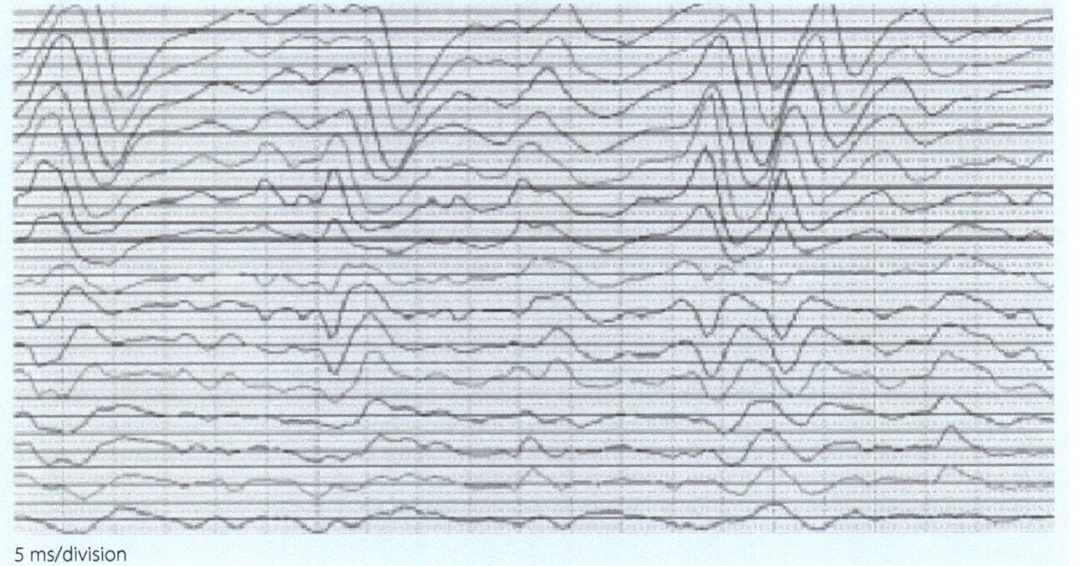

5 ms/division

## Lateral Deltoid

- **Anatomical landmark frames (ALF)**: A line between the acromion and the lateral epicondyle, above the deltoid tuberosity.
- **Experimental set up**: The subject was standing with one arm abducted at 45° and the elbow flexed. He or she then performed an isometric contraction during an abduction of the shoulder.
- **Optimal electrode site**: Between 0% and 17% or between 34% and 100% of the ALF.
- **Notes**: In 23 of the 40 subjects, an IZ was clearly detectable.

| Subjects investigated | IZs detected |
|---|---|
| 20 Males | 13 |
| 20 Females | 10 |

| Results | |
|---|---|
| Min | 17% |
| 1st quartile | 23% |
| Median | 28% |
| 3rd quartile | 30% |
| Max | 34% |

| Quality analysis | | | |
|---|---|---|---|
| | Items | Values | Score |
| **1** | Signal quality | 0 or 2 | 2 |
| **2** | Area without IZ | 0 or 2 | 2 |
| **3** | Physiological signal propagation | 0 or 1 | 1 |
| **4** | Motor units identification | 0 or 1 | 1 |
| | Total | | 6 |

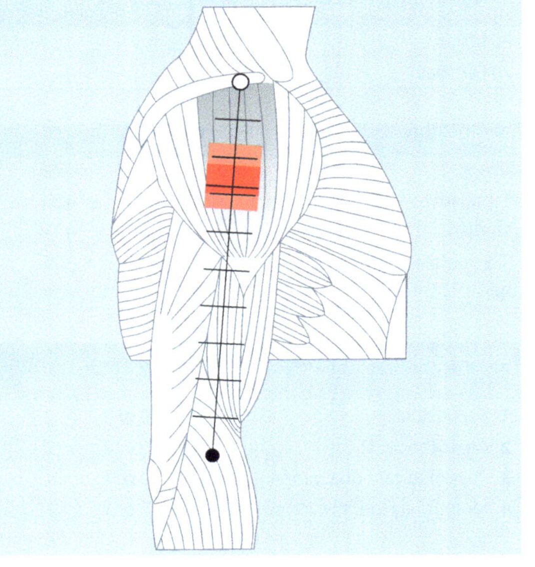

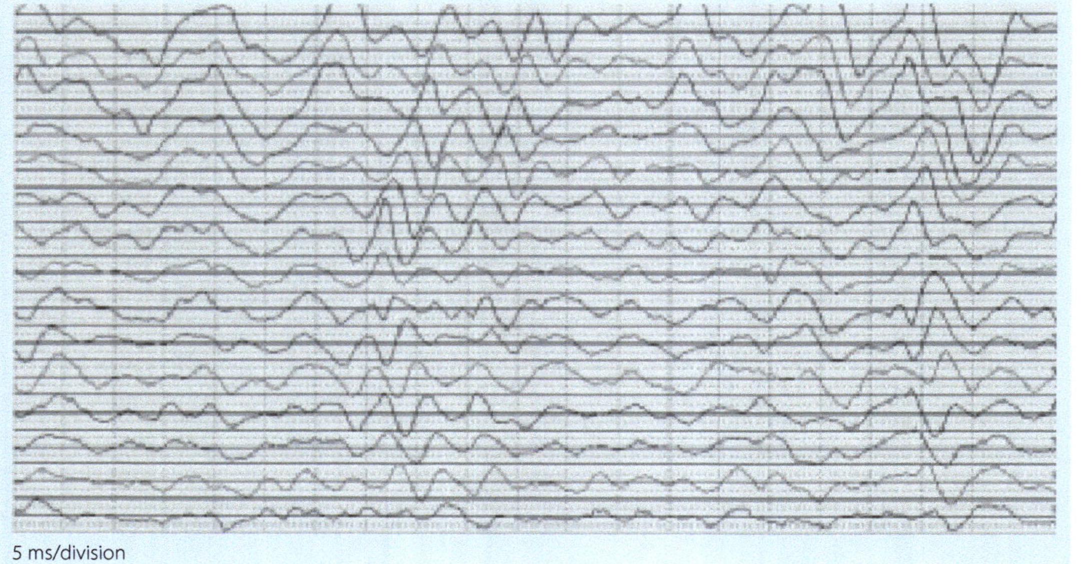

5 ms/division

# Anterior Deltoid

- **Anatomical landmark frames (ALF)**: A line between the coracoid process and the deltoid tuberosity.
- **Experimental set up**: The subject was standing with one arm along the body and the elbow flexed. He or she then performed an isometric contraction during an elevation of the arm.
- **Optimal electrode site**: Between 0% and 9% or between 67% and 100% of the ALF.
- **Notes**: In all 40 subjects, the propagation of motor unit action potentials was clearly seen.

| Subjects investigated | IZs detected |
|---|---|
| 20 Males | 20 |
| 20 Females | 20 |

| Results | |
|---|---|
| Min | 9% |
| 1st quartile | 19% |
| Median | 28% |
| 3rd quartile | 45% |
| Max | 67% |

| Quality analysis | | | |
|---|---|---|---|
| | **Items** | **Values** | **Score** |
| **1** | Signal quality | 0 or 2 | 2 |
| **2** | Area without IZ | 0 or 2 | 2 |
| **3** | Physiological signal propagation | 0 or 1 | 1 |
| **4** | Motor units identification | 0 or 1 | 1 |
| | Total | | 6 |

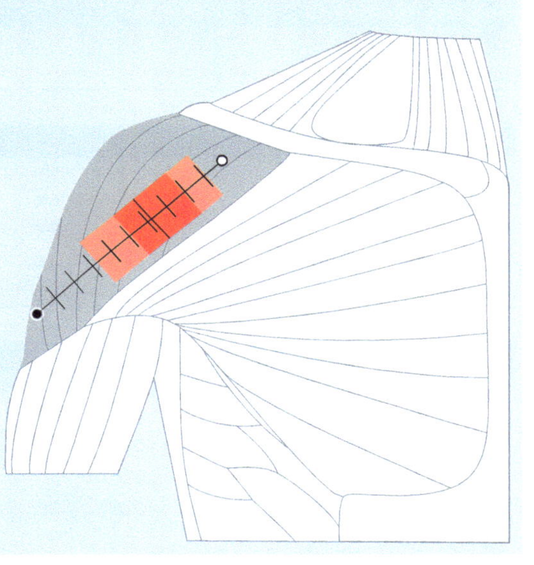

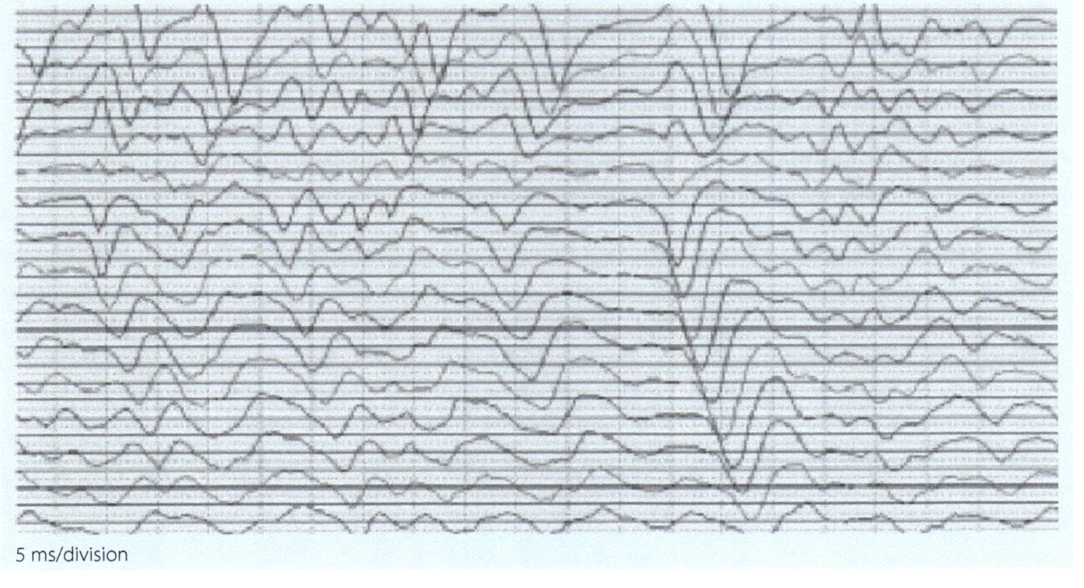

## Long Head of the Triceps

- **Anatomical landmark frames (ALF)**: The line between the angle of the acromion and the medial epicondyle.
- **Experimental set up**: The subject was standing with one arm along the body. He or she then performed an isometric contraction of the elbow starting with the elbow flexed at 45°.
- **Optimal electrode site**: On the muscle between 0% and 48% of the ALF. The probe was medially inclined with respect to the ALF.
- **Notes**: In 33 of the 40 subjects, the propagation of motor unit action potentials was clearly seen.

| Subjects investigated | IZs detected |
|---|---|
| 20 Males | 20 |
| 20 Females | 13 |

| Results | |
|---|---|
| Min | 48% |
| 1st quartile | 56% |
| Median | 58% |
| 3rd quartile | 63% |
| Max | 76% |

| Quality analysis | | | |
|---|---|---|---|
| | Items | Values | Score |
| **1** | Signal quality | 0 or 2 | 2 |
| **2** | Area without IZ | 0 or 2 | 2 |
| **3** | Physiological signal propagation | 0 or 1 | 1 |
| **4** | Motor units identification | 0 or 1 | 1 |
| | Total | | 6 |

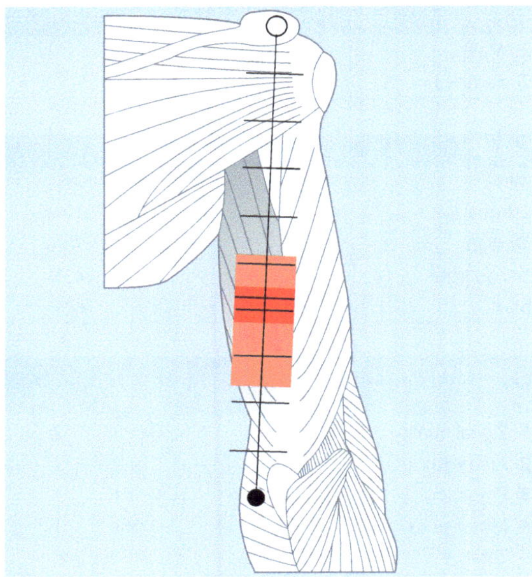

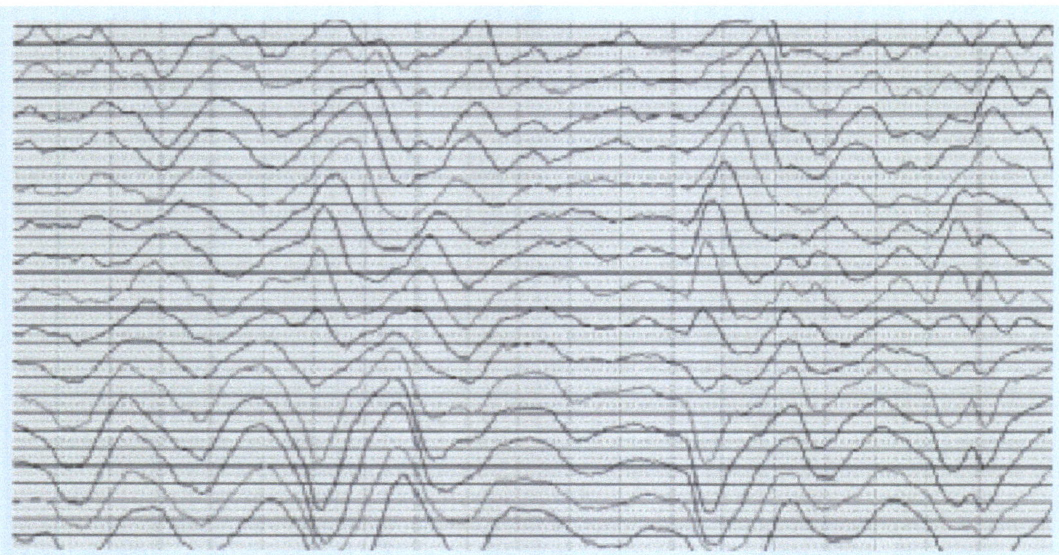

5 ms/division

## Lateral Head of the Triceps

- **Anatomical landmark frames (ALF)**: The line between the acromial angle and the lateral epicondyle.
- **Experimental set up**: The subject was standing with one arm along the body. He or she then performed an isometric contraction of the elbow starting with the elbow flexed at 45°.
- **Optimal electrode site**: On the muscle between 0% and 40% of the ALF or on the muscle belly between 66% and 100% of the ALF.
- **Notes**: In 37of the 40 subjects, the propagation of motor unit action potentials was clearly seen.

| Subjects investigated | IZs detected |
|---|---|
| 20 Males | 20 |
| 20 Females | 17 |

| Results | |
|---|---|
| Min | 40% |
| 1st quartile | 50% |
| Median | 53% |
| 3rd quartile | 59% |
| Max | 66% |

| Quality analysis | | |
|---|---|---|
| **Items** | **Values** | **Score** |
| **1** Signal quality | 0 or 2 | 2 |
| **2** Area without IZ | 0 or 2 | 2 |
| **3** Physiological signal propagation | 0 or 1 | 1 |
| **4** Motor units identification | 0 or 1 | 1 |
| Total | | 6 |

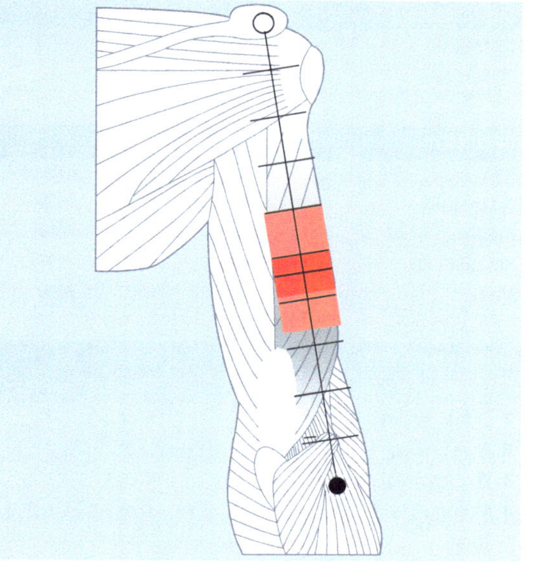

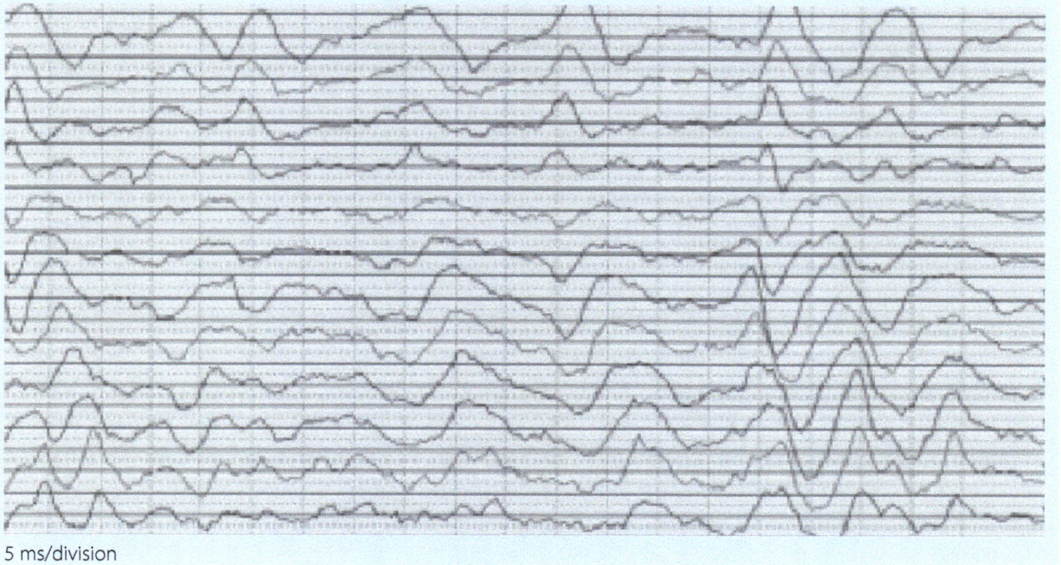

5 ms/division

# Short Head of the Biceps Brachii

- **Anatomical landmark frames (ALF)**: A line between the acromion and the distal insertion of the biceps brachii tendon.
- **Experimental set up**: The subject was seated on a chair with his or her right arm flexed at 90°. An isometric contraction was then performed. The probe was positioned medial to the ALF on the belly of the muscle.
- **Optimal electrode site**: On the muscle belly, before 61% of the ALF.
- **Notes**: In all 40 subjects, the propagation of motor unit action potentials was clearly seen. Nine subjects showed multiple innervation zones.

| Subjects investigated | IZs detected |
|---|---|
| 20 Males | 20 |
| 20 Females | 20 |

| Results | |
|---|---|
| Min | 61% |
| 1st quartile | 68% |
| Median | 70% |
| 3rd quartile | 74% |
| Max | 79% |

| Quality analysis | | |
|---|---|---|
| Items | Values | Score |
| **1** Signal quality | 0 or 2 | 2 |
| **2** Area without IZ | 0 or 2 | 2 |
| **3** Physiological signal propagation | 0 or 1 | 1 |
| **4** Motor units identification | 0 or 1 | 1 |
| Total | | 6 |

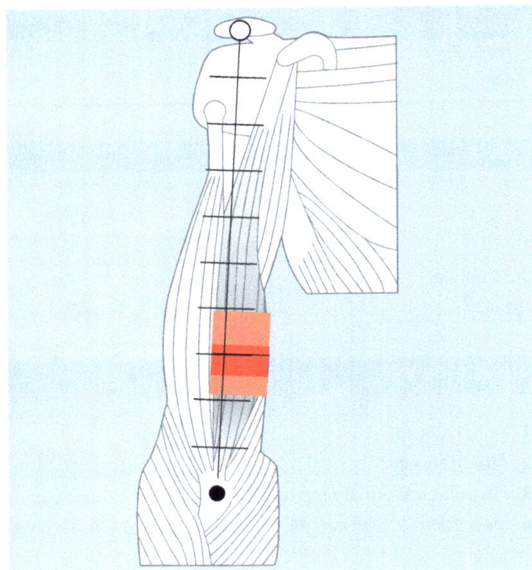

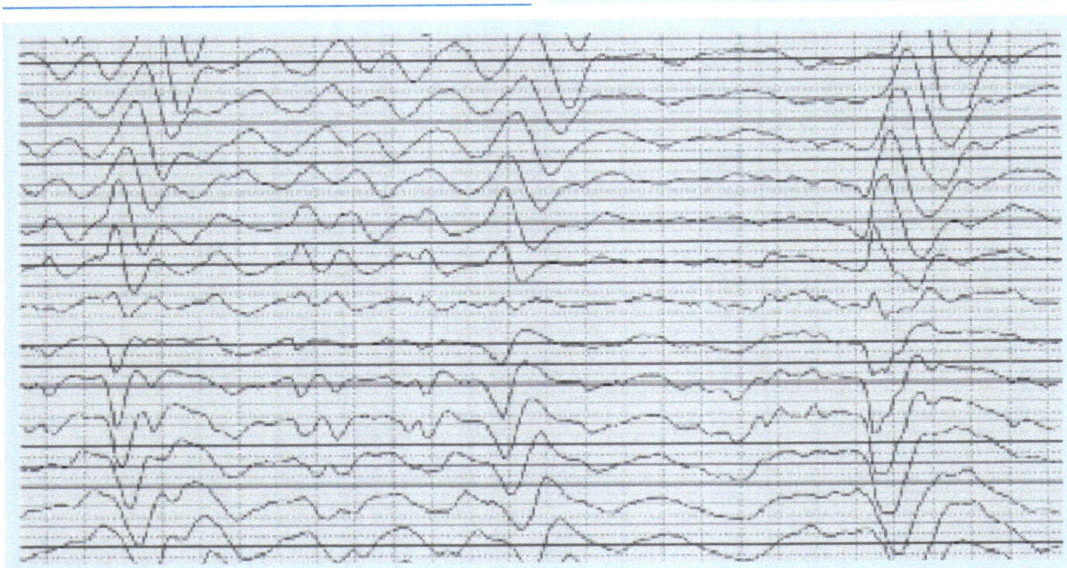

5 ms/division

## Long Head of the Biceps Brachii

- **Anatomical landmark frames (ALF)**: A line between the acromion and the distal insertion of the biceps brachii tendon.
- **Experimental set up**: The subject was seated on a chair with his or her right arm flexed at 90°. An isometric contraction was then performed during forearm flexion. The probe was positioned lateral to the ALF, on the belly of the muscle.
- **Optimal electrode site**: On the muscle belly, before 62% of the ALF.
- **Notes**: In all 40 subjects, the propagation of motor unit action potentials was clearly seen. Four subjects showed multiple innervation zones.

| Subjects investigated | IZs detected |
|---|---|
| 20 Males | 20 |
| 20 Females | 20 |

| Results | |
|---|---|
| Min | 62% |
| 1st quartile | 67% |
| Median | 70% |
| 3rd quartile | 74% |
| Max | 80% |

| Quality analysis | | | |
|---|---|---|---|
| | Items | Values | Score |
| 1 | Signal quality | 0 or 2 | 2 |
| 2 | Area without IZ | 0 or 2 | 2 |
| 3 | Physiological signal propagation | 0 or 1 | 1 |
| 4 | Motor units identification | 0 or 1 | 1 |
| | Total | | 6 |

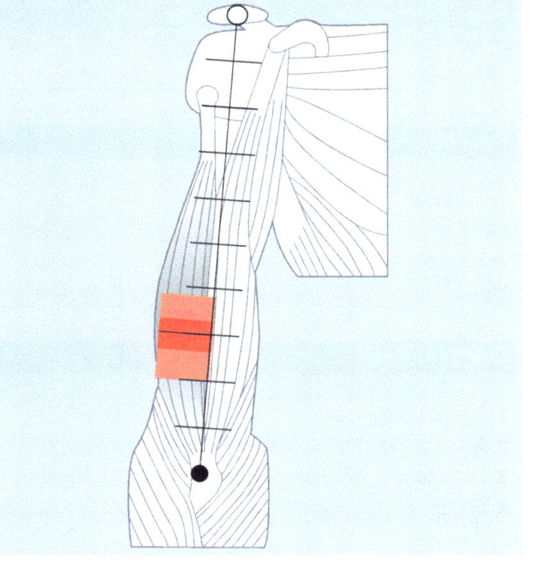

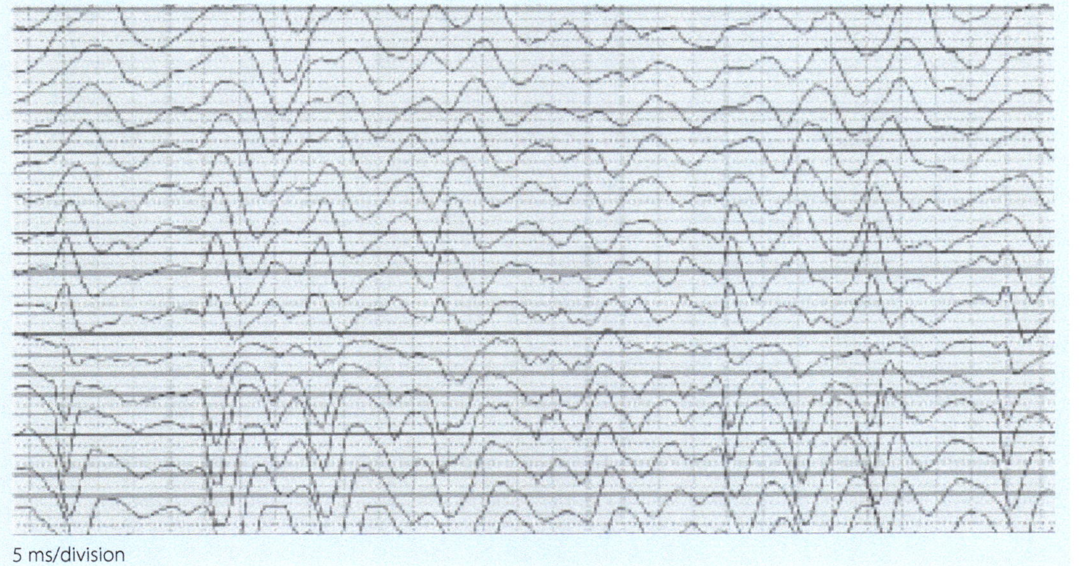

5 ms/division

# Palmaris Longus

- **Anatomical landmark frames (ALF)**: A line between the medial epicondyle and the distal end of the flexor retinaculum. The reference point at the flexor retinaculum is the tendon of the palmaris longus.
- **Experimental set up**: The subject was seated with the back erect, the elbow flexed at 90°, the forearm in complete supination, and the hand in the position as if holding several playing cards. He or she then performed an isometric contraction during flexion of the wrist against a resistance exerted at the hand.
- **Optimal electrode site**: Between 0% and 20% or between 47% and 100% of the ALF.

| Subjects investigated | IZs detected |
|---|---|
| 20 Males | 14 |
| 20 Females | 9 |

| Results | |
|---|---|
| Min | 20% |
| 1st quartile | 26% |
| Median | 30% |
| 3rd quartile | 37% |
| Max | 47% |

| Quality analysis | | |
|---|---|---|
| Items | Values | Score |
| **1** Signal quality | 0 or 2 | 2 |
| **2** Area without IZ | 0 or 2 | 2 |
| **3** Physiological signal propagation | 0 or 1 | 0 |
| **4** Motor units identification | 0 or 1 | 1 |
| Total | | 5 |

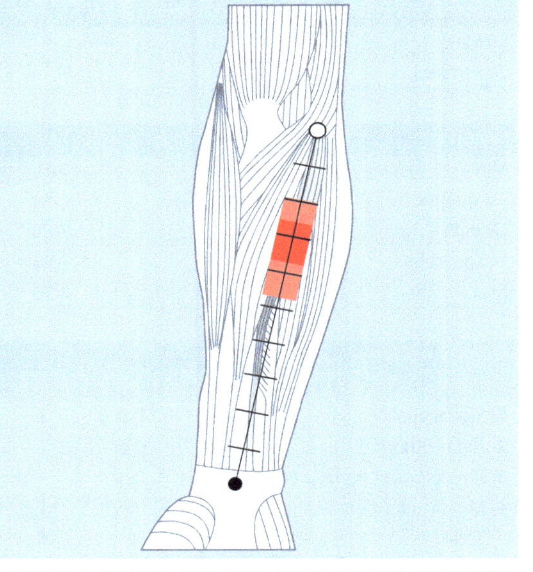

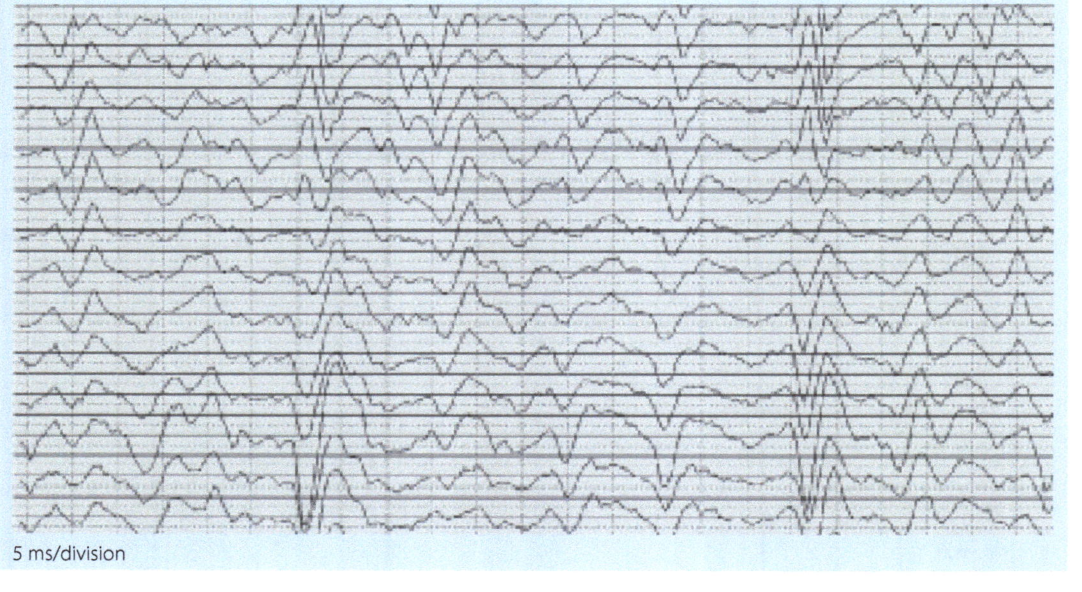

# Flexor Carpi Radialis

- **Anatomical landmark frames (ALF)**: A line from the medial epicondyle to the radial styloid process.
- **Experimental set up**: The subject was seated with the back erect, one elbow flexed at 90°, and the hand supinated. He or she then performed an isometric contraction during flexion of the wrist towards the radial side.
- **Optimal electrode site**: Between 0% and 13% or between 37% and 100% of the ALF.

| Subjects investigated | IZs detected |
|---|---|
| 20 Males | 15 |
| 20 Females | 13 |

| Results | |
|---|---|
| Min | 13% |
| 1st quartile | 26% |
| Median | 31% |
| 3rd quartile | 33% |
| Max | 37% |

| Quality analysis | | | |
|---|---|---|---|
| | Items | Values | Score |
| **1** | Signal quality | 0 or 2 | 2 |
| **2** | Area without IZ | 0 or 2 | 2 |
| **3** | Physiological signal propagation | 0 or 1 | 0 |
| **4** | Motor units identification | 0 or 1 | 1 |
| | Total | | 5 |

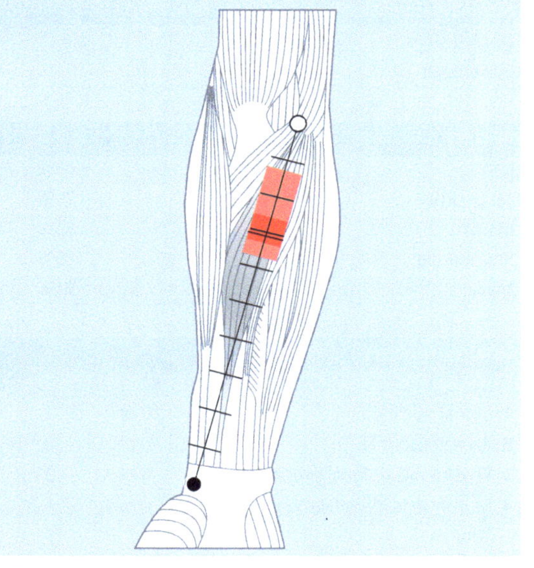

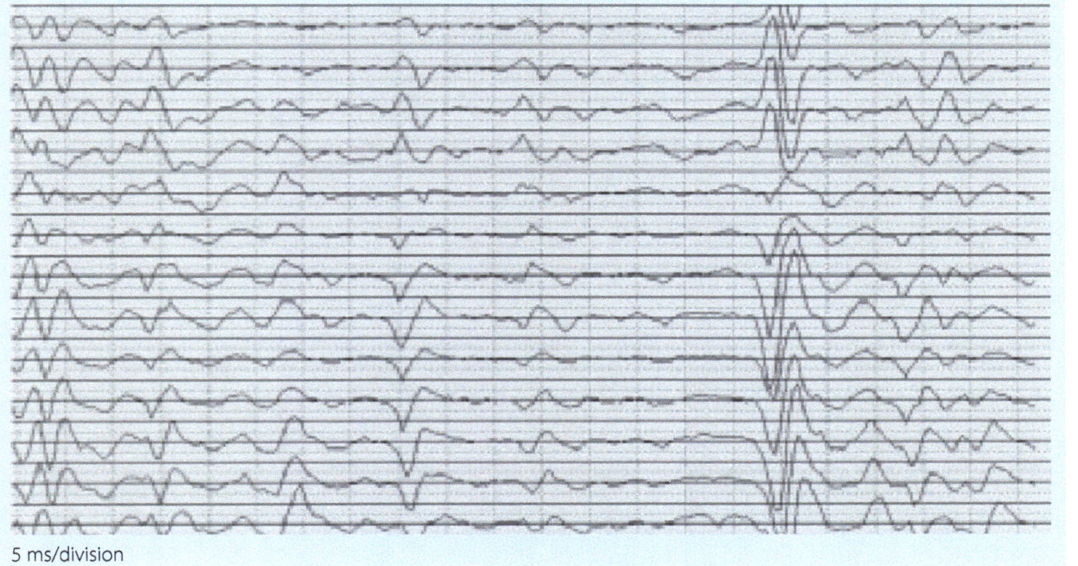

5 ms/division

# Pronator Teres

- **Anatomical landmark frames (ALF)**: A line between the medial epicondyle and the origin of the biceps brachii tendon.
- **Experimental set up**: The subject was seated with the back erect, the arm flexed at 90°, and the forearm supinated. He or she then performed an isometric contraction during pronation of the forearm.
- **Optimal electrode site**: Between 0% and 67% of the ALF.
- **Notes**: All 40 subjects showed clear motor unit action potentials propagation. Nine subjects showed multiple IZs.

| Subjects investigated | IZs detected |
|---|---|
| 20 Males | 11 |
| 20 Females | 9 |

| Results | |
|---|---|
| Min | 67% |
| 1st quartile | 79% |
| Median | 85% |
| 3rd quartile | 88% |
| Max | 91% |

| Quality analysis | | | |
|---|---|---|---|
| | Items | Values | Score |
| **1** | Signal quality | 0 or 2 | 2 |
| **2** | Area without IZ | 0 or 2 | 2 |
| **3** | Physiological signal propagation | 0 or 1 | 0 |
| **4** | Motor units identification | 0 or 1 | 1 |
| | Total | | 5 |

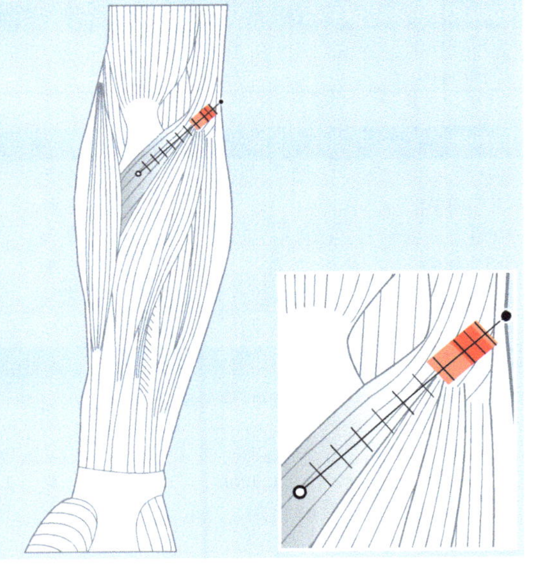

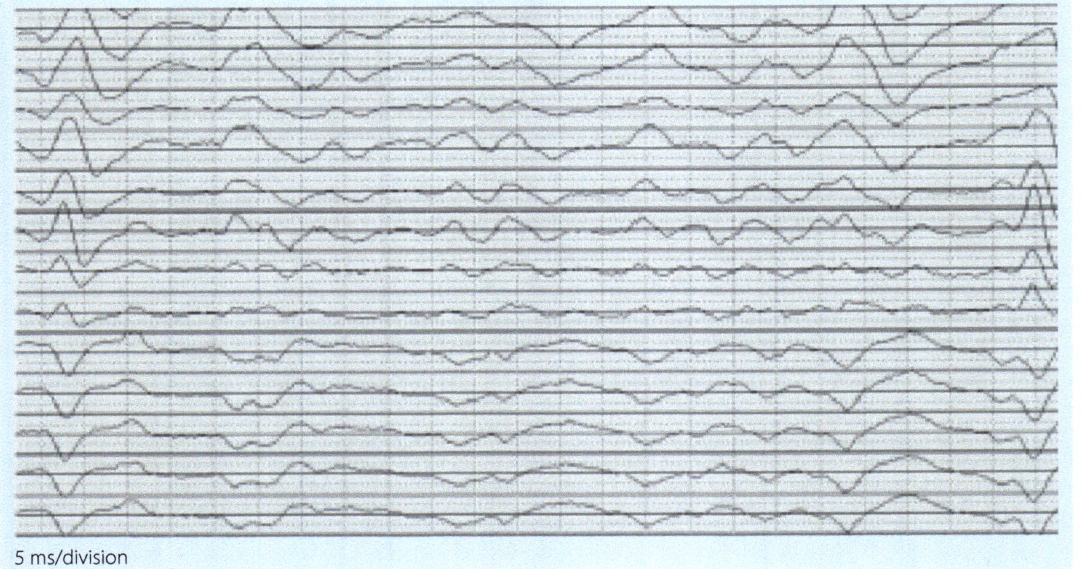

5 ms/division

# Brachioradialis

- **Anatomical landmark frames (ALF)**: A line from the styloid process to a midpoint on the line between the lateral and medial epicondyles.
- **Experimental set up**: The subject was seated with the forearm flexed at 90° in neutral position. He or she then performed an isometric contraction during flexion of the forearm.
- **Optimal electrode site**: Between 32% and 100% of the ALF.
- **Notes**: In case of a distal positioning of the electrode, the muscle belly is located proximally.

| Subjects investigated | IZs detected |
|---|---|
| 20 Males | 20 |
| 20 Females | 20 |

| Results | |
|---|---|
| Min | 7% |
| 1st quartile | 11% |
| Median | 17% |
| 3rd quartile | 27% |
| Max | 32% |

| Quality analysis | | | |
|---|---|---|---|
| | Items | Values | Score |
| 1 | Signal quality | 0 or 2 | 2 |
| 2 | Area without IZ | 0 or 2 | 2 |
| 3 | Physiological signal propagation | 0 or 1 | 1 |
| 4 | Motor units identification | 0 or 1 | 1 |
| | Total | | 6 |

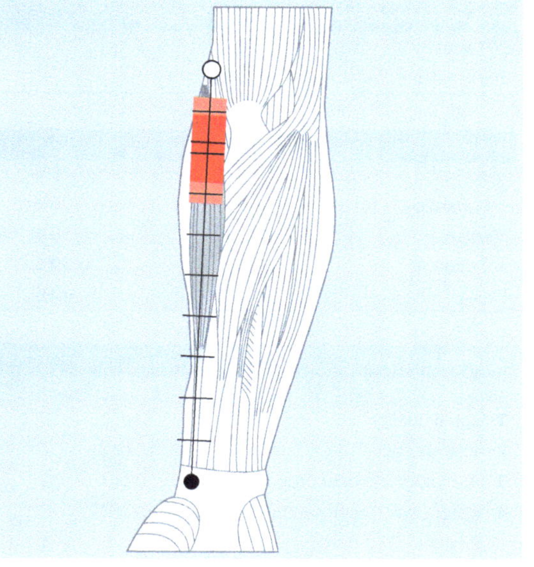

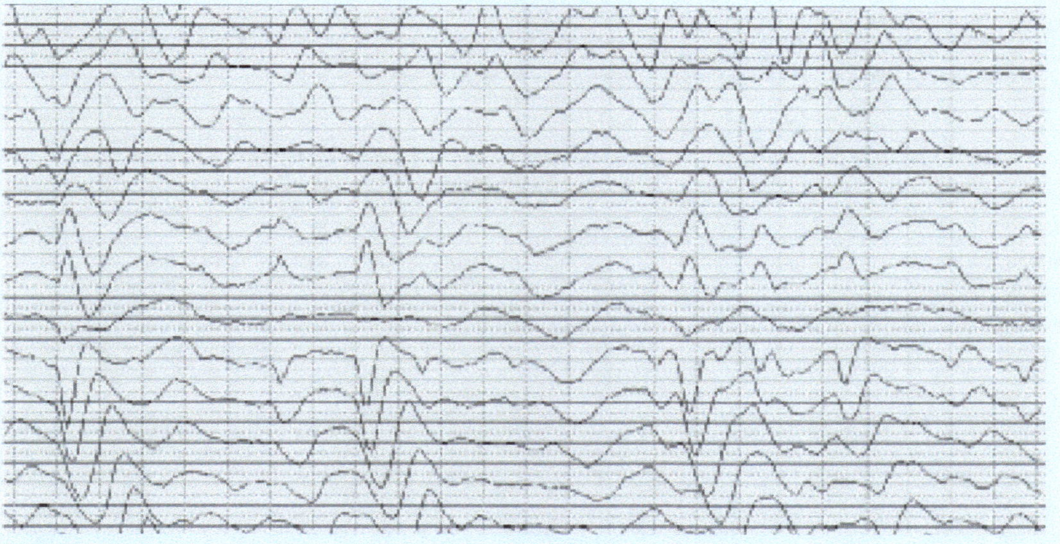

5 ms/division

## Extensor Carpi Ulnaris

- **Anatomical landmark frames (ALF)**: A line between the lateral epicondyle and the styloid process of the ulna.
- **Experimental set up**: The subject was seated with elbow flexed at 90° and the forearm in complete pronation. He or she then performed an isometric contraction during extension of the wrist towards the ulnar side.
- **Optimal electrode site**: Not applicable.
- **Notes**: IZs were detected only exceptionally.

| Subjects investigated | IZs detected |
|---|---|
| 20 Males | 1 |
| 20 Females | 2 |

| Results | |
|---|---|
| Min | 13% |
| 1st quartile | 26% |
| Median | 38% |
| 3rd quartile | 39% |
| Max | 39% |

| Quality analysis | | | |
|---|---|---|---|
| | Items | Values | Score |
| **1** | Signal quality | 0 or 2 | 2 |
| **2** | Area without IZ | 0 or 2 | 2 |
| **3** | Physiological signal propagation | 0 or 1 | 0 |
| **4** | Motor units identification | 0 or 1 | 0 |
| | Total | | 4 |

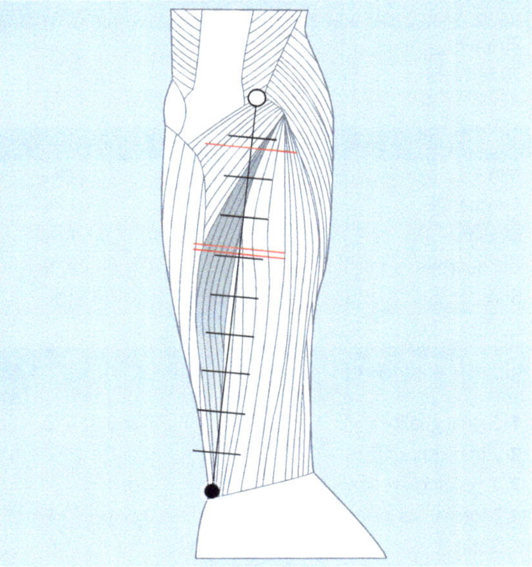

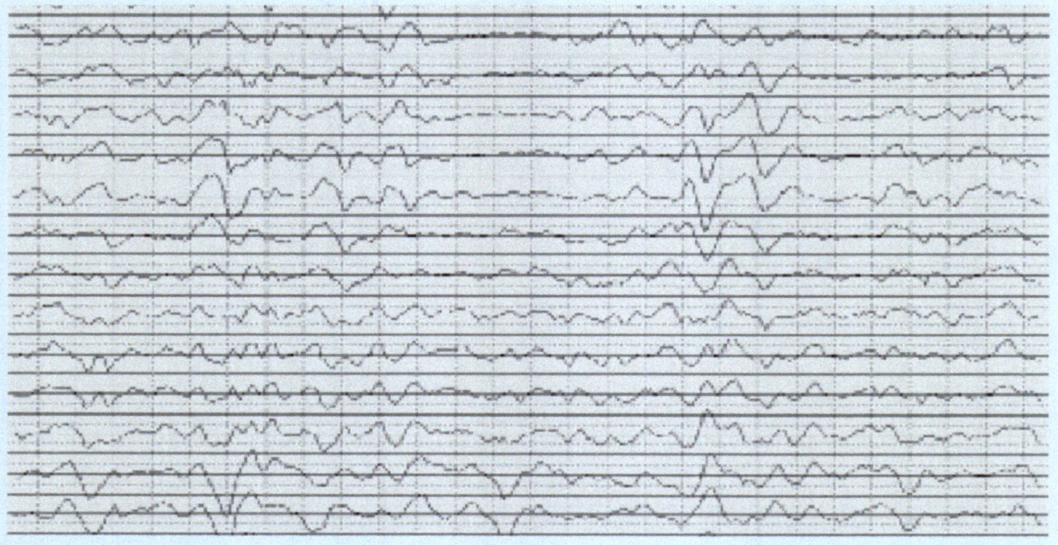

5 ms/division

## Extensor Carpi Radialis

- **Anatomical landmark frames (ALF)**: A line from the midpoint between the radial and ulnar styloid processes to the lateral supracondylar ridge.
- **Experimental set up**: The subject was seated with one elbow flexed at 90° and the forearm in complete pronation. He or she then performed an isometric contraction during extension of the wrist towards the radial side.
- **Optimal electrode site**: Between 0% and 17% or between 42% and 100% of the ALF.

| Subjects investigated | IZs detected |
|---|---|
| 20 Males | 7 |
| 20 Females | 14 |

| Results | |
|---|---|
| Min | 17% |
| 1st quartile | 27% |
| Median | 34% |
| 3rd quartile | 38% |
| Max | 42% |

| Quality analysis | | | |
|---|---|---|---|
| | Items | Values | Score |
| 1 | Signal quality | 0 or 2 | 2 |
| 2 | Area without IZ | 0 or 2 | 2 |
| 3 | Physiological signal propagation | 0 or 1 | 0 |
| 4 | Motor units identification | 0 or 1 | 1 |
| | Total | | 5 |

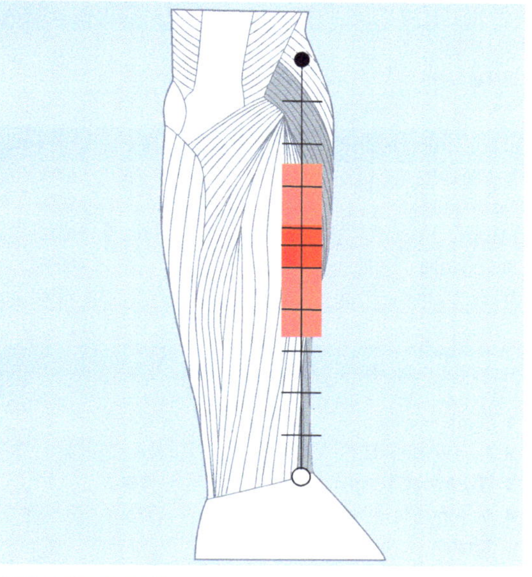

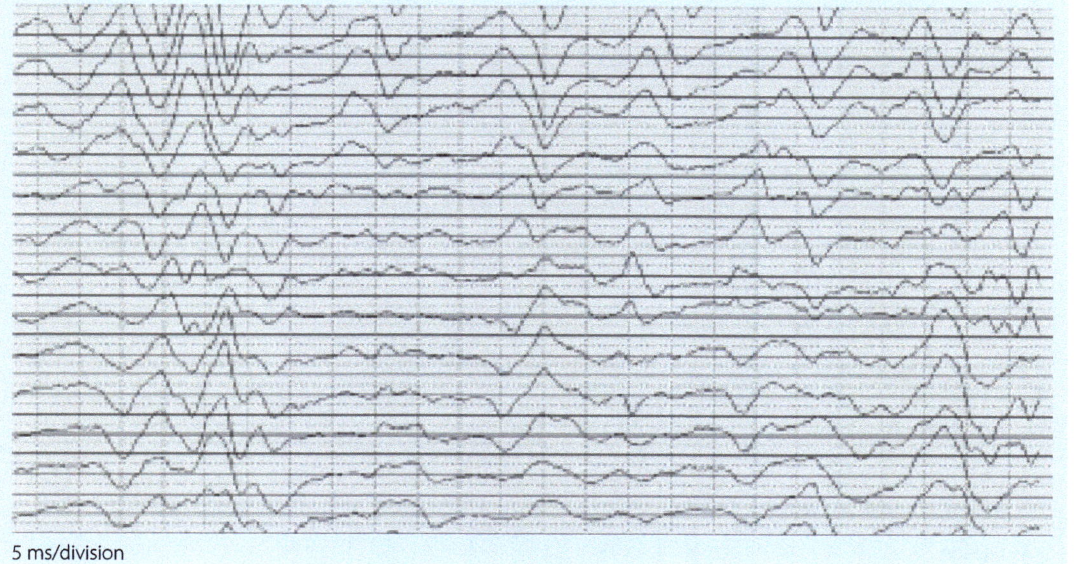

5 ms/division

# Abductor Digiti Minimi

- **Anatomical landmark frames (ALF)**: A line between the pisiform bone and the base of the fifth metacarpal bone.
- **Experimental set up**: The subject was seated with the back erect, the elbow flexed at 90°, and the hand supinated. He or she then performed an isometric contraction during a pure abduction of the fifth finger.
- **Optimal electrode site**: Between 0% and 42% or between 75% and 100% of the ALF.

| Subjects investigated | IZs detected |
|---|---|
| 20 Males | 20 |
| 20 Females | 20 |

| Results | |
|---|---|
| Min | 42% |
| 1st quartile | 58% |
| Median | 65% |
| 3rd quartile | 69% |
| Max | 75% |

| Quality analysis | | | |
|---|---|---|---|
| | Items | Values | Score |
| 1 | Signal quality | 0 or 2 | 2 |
| 2 | Area without IZ | 0 or 2 | 2 |
| 3 | Physiological signal propagation | 0 or 1 | 1 |
| 4 | Motor units identification | 0 or 1 | 1 |
| | Total | | 6 |

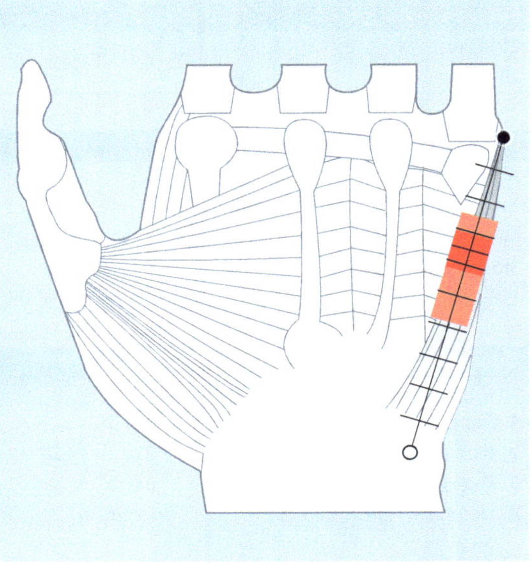

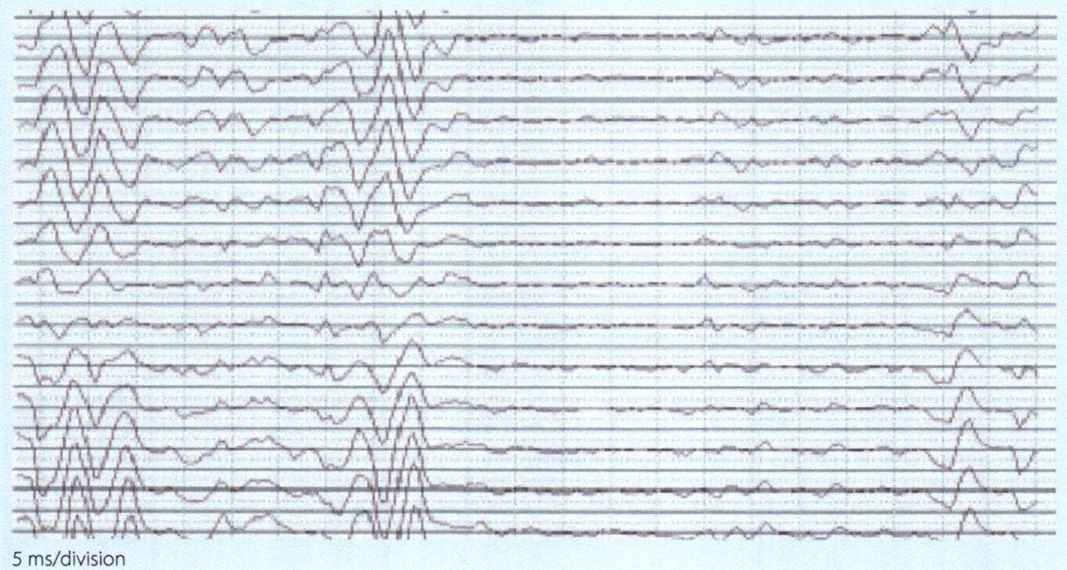

5 ms/division

# Flexor Pollicis Brevis

- **Anatomical landmark frames (ALF)**: The midpoint between the radial and ulnar styloid processes is marked on the skin. Also, 1/3 of the distance between this point and the base of the middle fingers is marked on the skin. Finally, the ALF is drawn between this point and the base of the proximal phalanx of the thumb.
- **Experimental set up**: The subject was seated with the back erect, the forearm flexed at 90°, and the hand in neutral position. He or she then performed an isometric contraction during pure flexion against resistance exerted at the base of the finger.
- **Optimal electrode site**: After 59% of the ALF.

| Subjects investigated | IZs detected |
|---|---|
| 20 Males | 20 |
| 20 Females | 20 |

| Results | |
|---|---|
| Min | 19% |
| 1st quartile | 28% |
| Median | 40% |
| 3rd quartile | 45% |
| Max | 59% |

| Quality analysis | | | |
|---|---|---|---|
| | Items | Values | Score |
| 1 | Signal quality | 0 or 2 | 2 |
| 2 | Area without IZ | 0 or 2 | 2 |
| 3 | Physiological signal propagation | 0 or 1 | 1 |
| 4 | Motor units identification | 0 or 1 | 1 |
| | Total | | 6 |

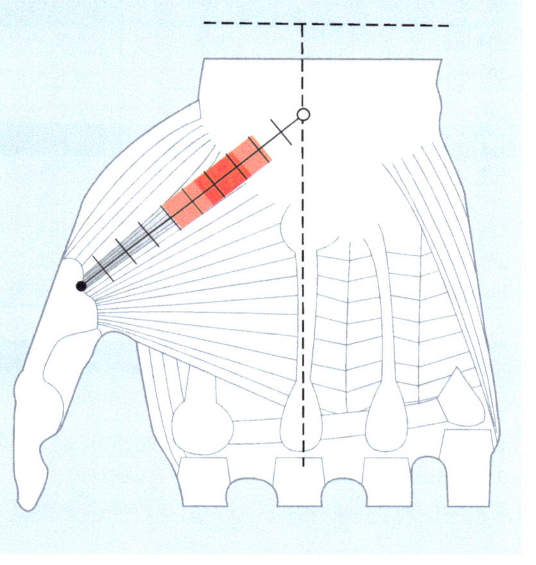

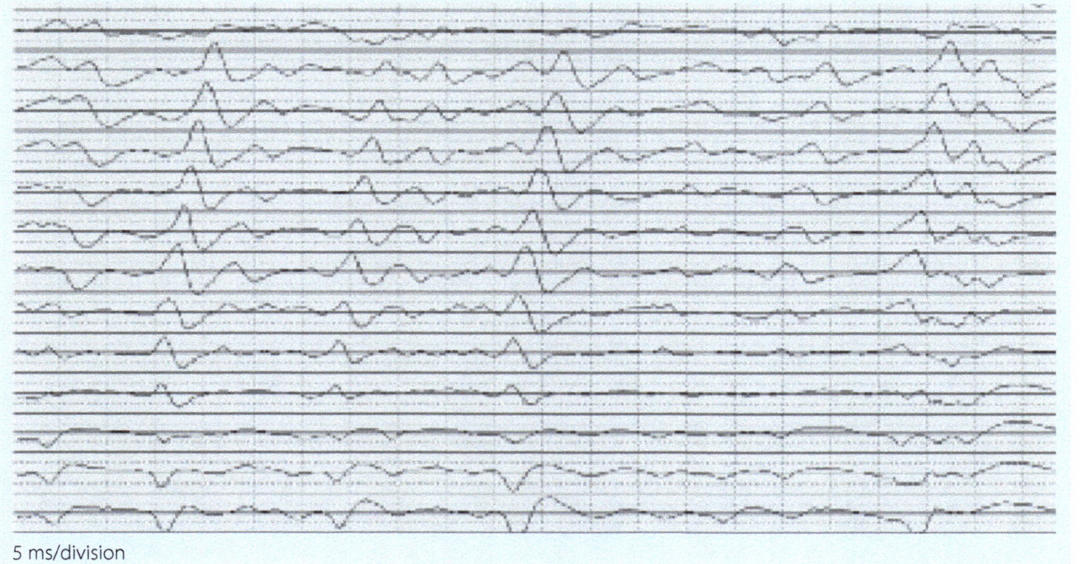

5 ms/division

# Abductor Pollicis Brevis

- **Anatomical landmark frames (ALF)**: A line between the tubercle of the scaphoid bone and the base of the first metacarpal bone.
- **Experimental set up**: The subject was seated with the back erect, the forearm flexed at 90°, and the hand in neutral position. He or she then performed an isometric contraction during a pure abduction of the thumb against the base of the first metacarpal.
- **Optimal electrode site**: Between 0% and 35% or between 62% and 100% of the ALF.

| Subjects investigated | IZs detected |
|---|---|
| 20 Males | 18 |
| 20 Females | 18 |

| Results | |
|---|---|
| Min | 35% |
| 1st quartile | 46% |
| Median | 49% |
| 3rd quartile | 53% |
| Max | 62% |

| Quality analysis | | |
|---|---|---|
| Items | Values | Score |
| **1** Signal quality | 0 or 2 | 2 |
| **2** Area without IZ | 0 or 2 | 2 |
| **3** Physiological signal propagation | 0 or 1 | 1 |
| **4** Motor units identification | 0 or 1 | 1 |
| Total | | 6 |

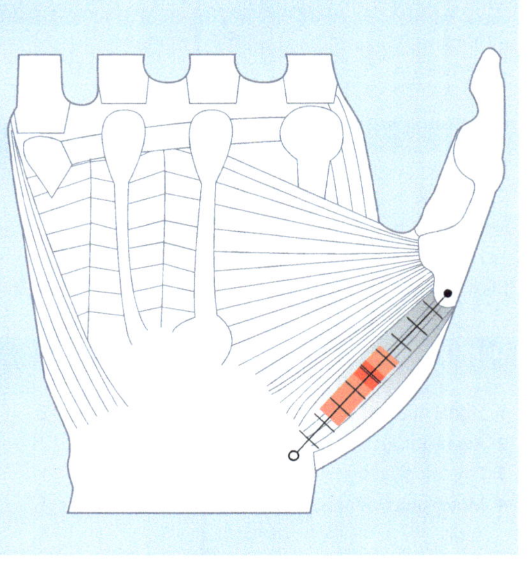

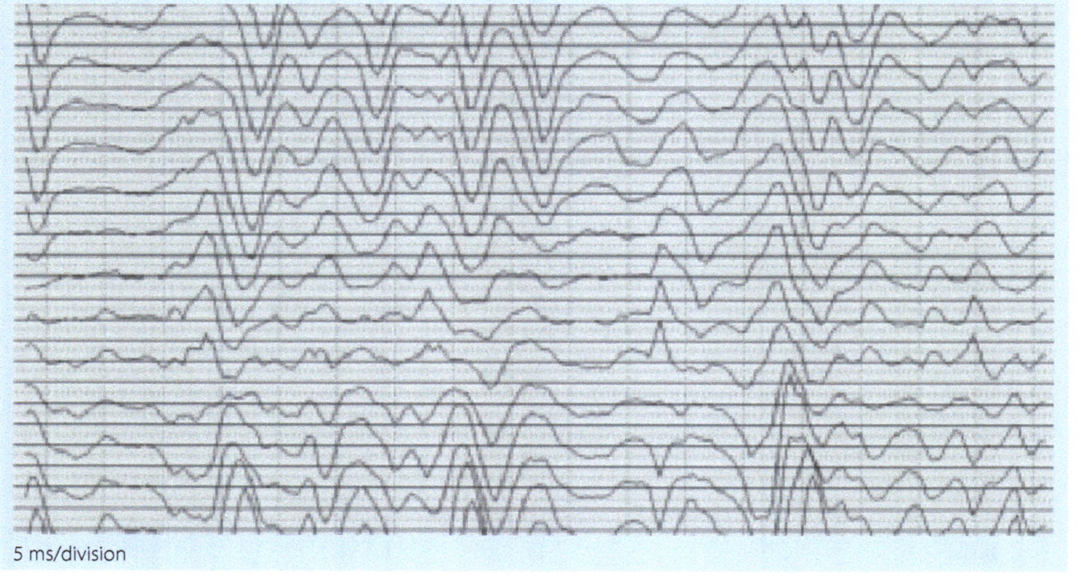

# Lower Limb

## Gluteus Maximus

- **Anatomical landmark frames (ALF)**: A line between S2 and the greater trochanter.
- **Experimental set up**: The subject was seated with one knee flexed at 90°. He or she then performed an isometric contraction during hip extension.
- **Optimal electrode site**: Between 0% and 22% or between 49% and 100% of the ALF.

| Subjects investigated | IZs detected |
|---|---|
| 20 Males | 14 |
| 20 Females | 13 |

| Results | |
|---|---|
| Min | 22% |
| 1st quartile | 36% |
| Median | 40% |
| 3rd quartile | 42% |
| Max | 49% |

| Quality analysis | | | |
|---|---|---|---|
| | Items | Values | Score |
| 1 | Signal quality | 0 or 2 | 2 |
| 2 | Area without IZ | 0 or 2 | 2 |
| 3 | Physiological signal propagation | 0 or 1 | 0 |
| 4 | Motor units identification | 0 or 1 | 0 |
| | Total | | 4 |

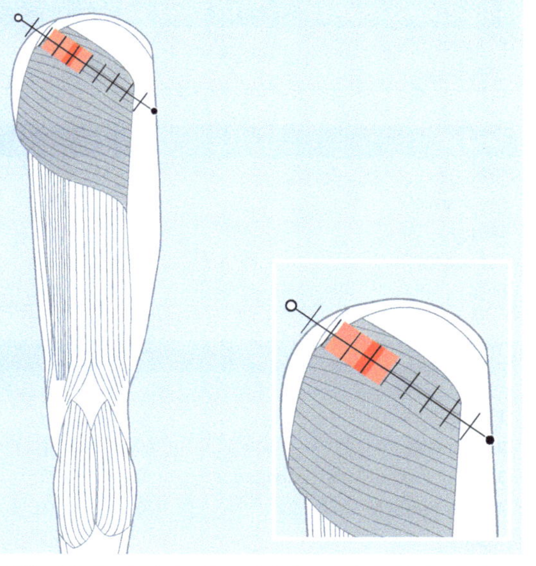

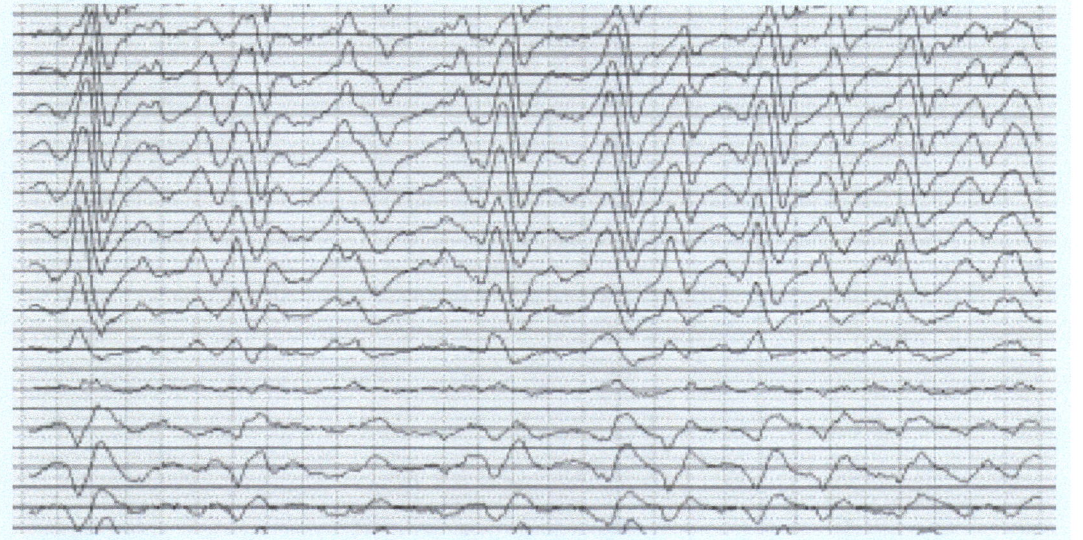

5 ms/division

## Gluteus Medius

- **Anatomical landmark frames (ALF)**: A line between the greater trochanter and the highest point of the iliac crest.
- **Experimental set up**: The subjects lay on his or her side. An isometric contraction was then performed during an abduction of the hip placed neutrally with respect to flexion, extension, and rotation.
- **Optimal electrode site**: Between 0% and 26% or between 55% and 100% of the ALF.

| Subjects investigated | IZs detected |
|---|---|
| 20 Males | 7 |
| 20 Females | 3 |

| Results | |
|---|---|
| Min | 26% |
| 1st quartile | 34% |
| Median | 45% |
| 3rd quartile | 51% |
| Max | 55% |

| Quality analysis | | |
|---|---|---|
| **Items** | **Values** | **Score** |
| **1** Signal quality | 0 or 2 | 0 |
| **2** Area without IZ | 0 or 2 | 2 |
| **3** Physiological signal propagation | 0 or 1 | 0 |
| **4** Motor units identification | 0 or 1 | 1 |
| Total | | 3 |

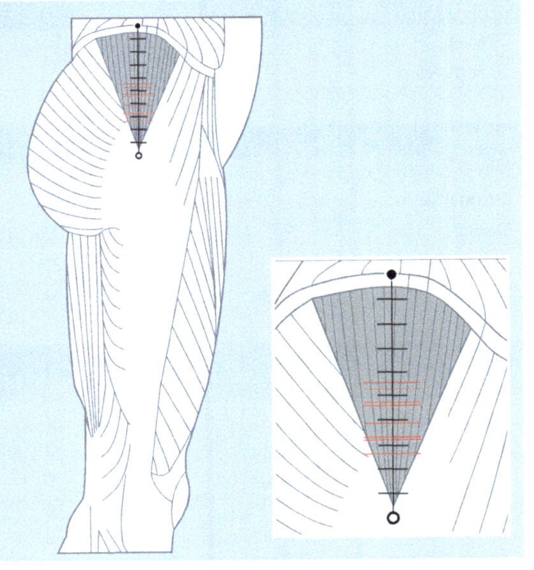

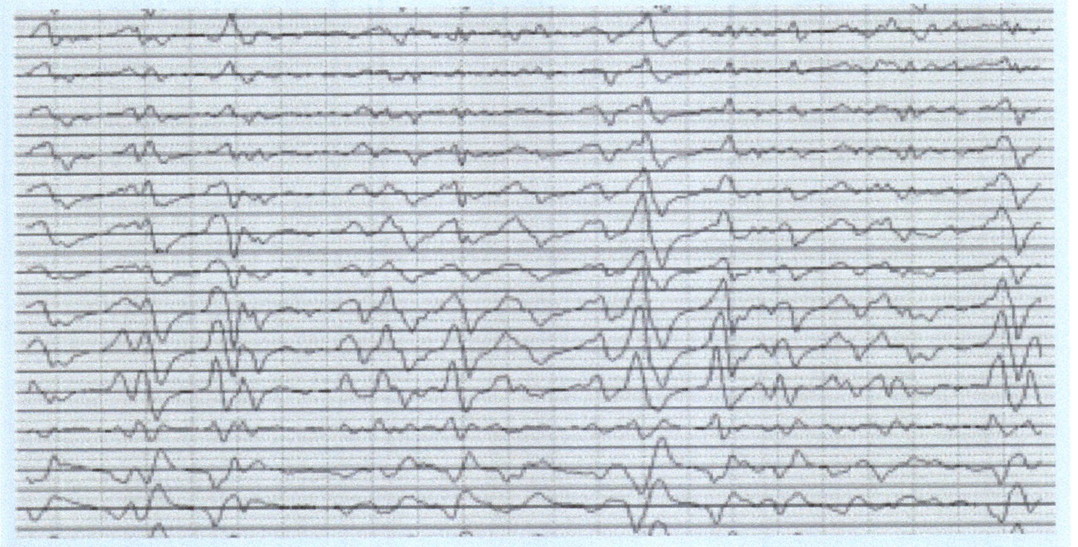

5 ms/division

# Semitendinosus

- **Anatomical landmark frames (ALF)**: A line between the ischial tuberosity and the medial side of the popliteal cavity.
- **Experimental set up**: The subject was prone with one knee flexed at 45°. He or she then performed an isometric contraction during flexion of the knee placed in internal rotation.
- **Optimal electrode site**: Between 0% and 26% or between 74% and 100% of the ALF.

| Subjects investigated | IZs detected |
|---|---|
| 20 Males | 11 |
| 20 Females | 9 |

| Results | |
|---|---|
| Min | 26% |
| 1st quartile | 31% |
| Median | 39% |
| 3rd quartile | 42% |
| Max | 52% |

| Quality analysis | | | |
|---|---|---|---|
| | Items | Values | Score |
| **1** | Signal quality | 0 or 2 | 2 |
| **2** | Area without IZ | 0 or 2 | 2 |
| **3** | Physiological signal propagation | 0 or 1 | 0 |
| **4** | Motor units identification | 0 or 1 | 1 |
| | Total | | 5 |

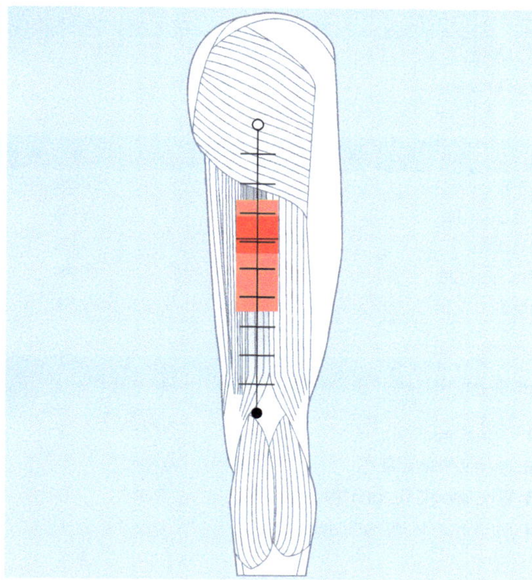

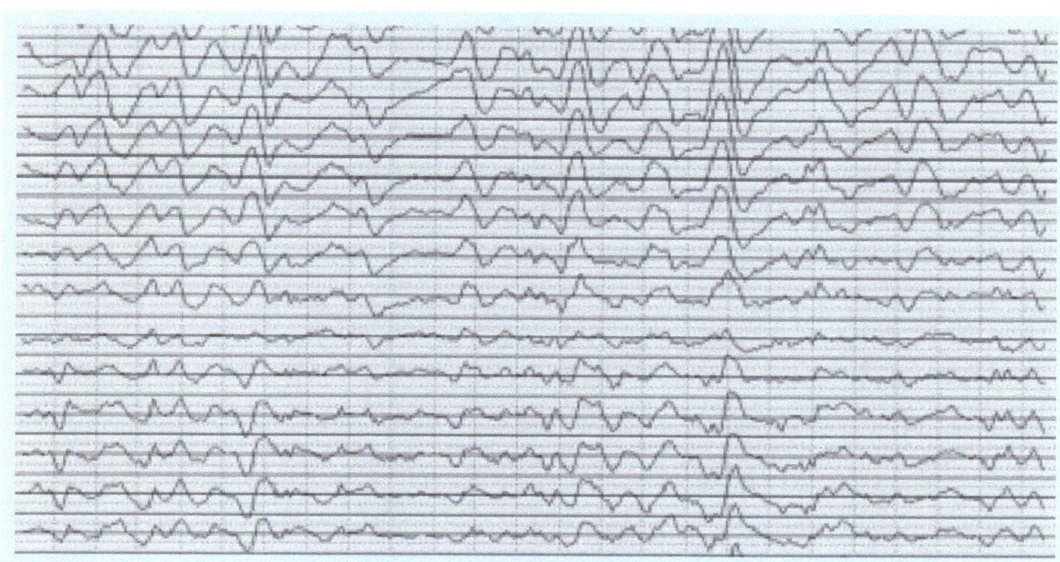

5 ms/division

## Biceps Femoris

- **Anatomical landmark frames (ALF)**: A line between the ischial tuberosity and the lateral side of the popliteal cavity.
- **Experimental set up**: The subject was prone with the knee flexed at 45°. He or she then performed an isometric contraction during flexion of the knee placed in external rotation.
- **Optimal electrode site**: On the muscle belly between 0% and 22% or between 72% and 100% of the ALF.

| Subjects investigated | IZs detected |
|---|---|
| 20 Males | 12 |
| 20 Females | 8 |

| Results | |
|---|---|
| Min | 22% |
| 1st quartile | 31% |
| Median | 51% |
| 3rd quartile | 63% |
| Max | 72% |

| Quality analysis | | | |
|---|---|---|---|
| | Items | Values | Score |
| 1 | Signal quality | 0 or 2 | 2 |
| 2 | Area without IZ | 0 or 2 | 2 |
| 3 | Physiological signal propagation | 0 or 1 | 0 |
| 4 | Motor units identification | 0 or 1 | 1 |
| | Total | | 5 |

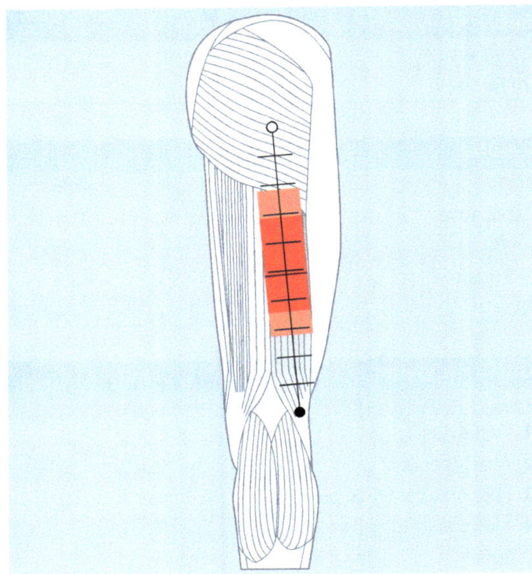

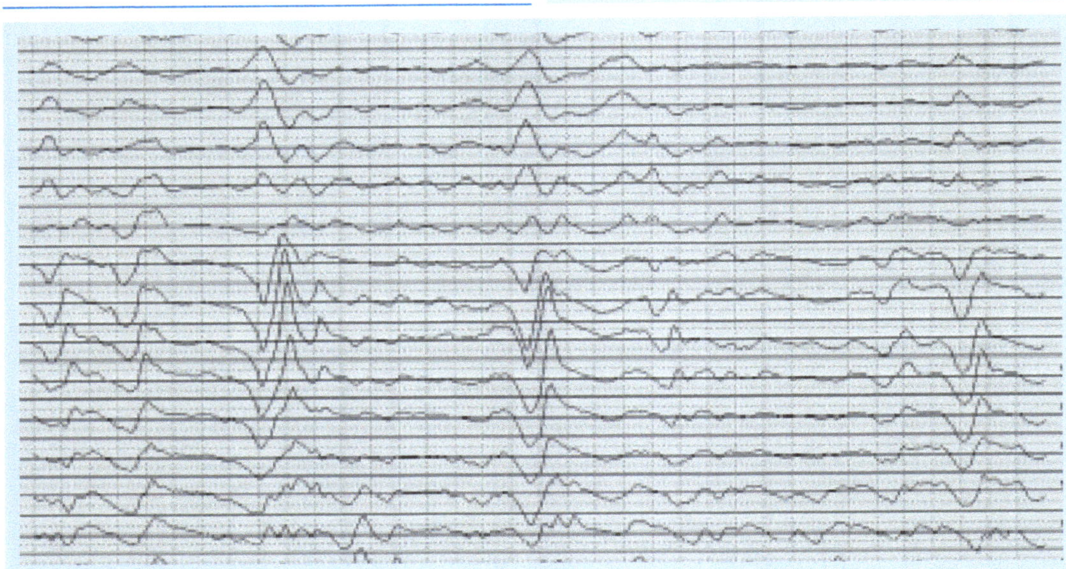

5 ms/division

## Gastrocnemius Medialis

- **Anatomical landmark frames (ALF)**: A line between the medial side of the Achilles tendon insertion and the medial side of the popliteal cavity.
- **Experimental set up**: A line between the medial side of the Achilles tendon insertion and the medial side of the popliteal cavity.
- **Optimal electrode site**: Between 87% and 100% of the ALF.

| Subjects investigated | IZs detected |
|---|---|
| 20 Males | 12 |
| 20 Females | 8 |

| Results | |
|---|---|
| Min | 53% |
| 1st quartile | 60% |
| Median | 66% |
| 3rd quartile | 71% |
| Max | 87% |

| Quality analysis | | | |
|---|---|---|---|
| | **Items** | **Values** | **Score** |
| **1** | Signal quality | 0 or 2 | 2 |
| **2** | Area without IZ | 0 or 2 | 2 |
| **3** | Physiological signal propagation | 0 or 1 | 0 |
| **4** | Motor units identification | 0 or 1 | 1 |
| | Total | | 5 |

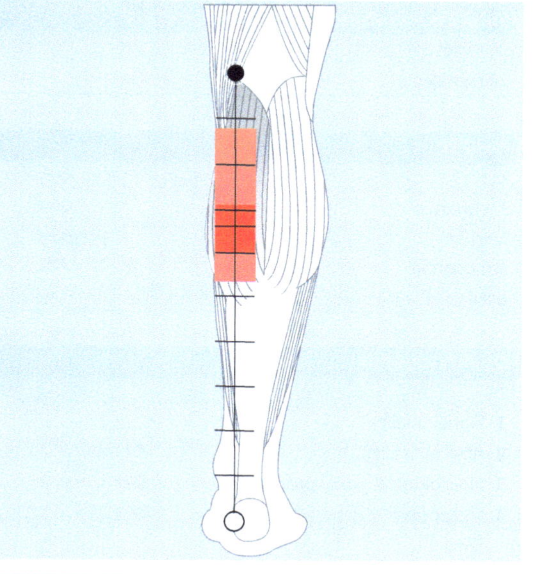

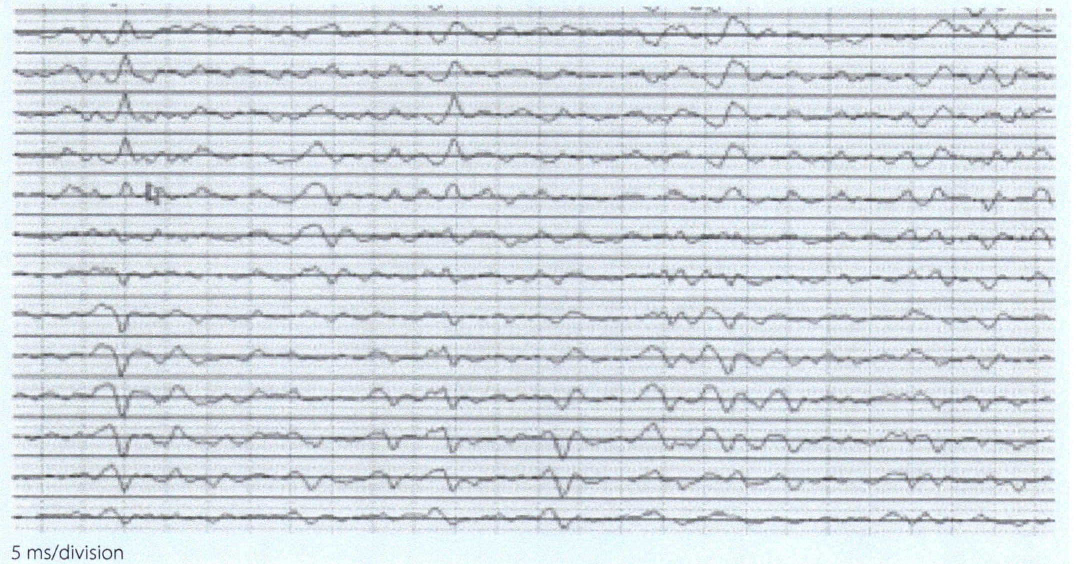

5 ms/division

## Gastrocnemius Lateralis

- **Anatomical landmark frames (ALF)**: A line between the lateral side of the Achilles tendon insertion and the lateral side of the popliteal cavity.
- **Experimental set up**: The subject was prone with the knee extended. He or she then performed an isometric contraction during plantar flexion of the ankle.
- **Optimal electrode site**: Between 75% and 100% of the ALF.

| Subjects investigated | IZs detected |
|---|---|
| 20 Males | 9 |
| 20 Females | 5 |

| Results | |
|---|---|
| Min | 60% |
| 1st quartile | 64% |
| Median | 65% |
| 3rd quartile | 72% |
| Max | 75% |

| Quality analysis | | | |
|---|---|---|---|
| | Items | Values | Score |
| 1 | Signal quality | 0 or 2 | 2 |
| 2 | Area without IZ | 0 or 2 | 2 |
| 3 | Physiological signal propagation | 0 or 1 | 0 |
| 4 | Motor units identification | 0 or 1 | 1 |
| | Total | | 5 |

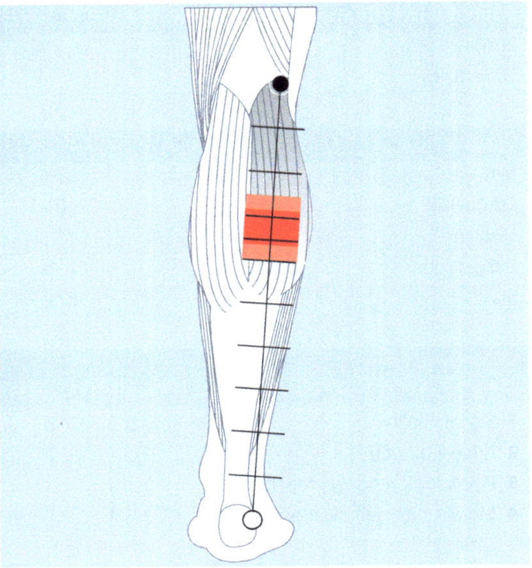

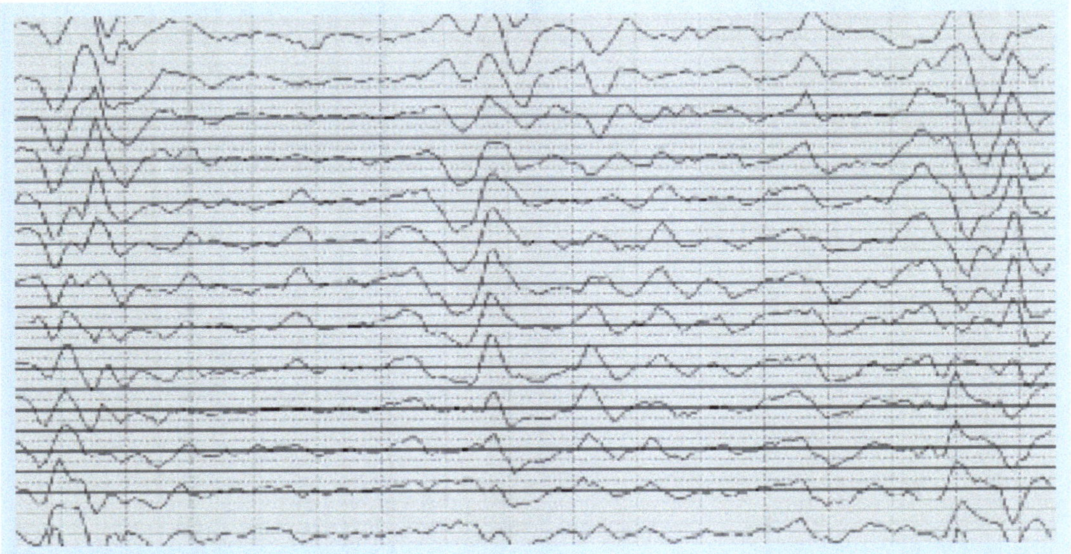

5 ms/division

## Soleus

- **Anatomical landmark frames (ALF)**: A line between the medial side of the Achilles tendon insertion and the head of the fibula.
- **Experimental set up**: The subject was prone with one knee bent at 20°. He or she then performed an isometric contraction during plantar flexion of the ankle.
- **Optimal electrode site**: Between 0 and 32% of ALF.

| Subjects investigated | IZs detected |
|---|---|
| 20 Males | 7 |
| 20 Females | 4 |

| Results | |
|---|---|
| Min | 32% |
| 1st quartile | 39% |
| Median | 42% |
| 3rd quartile | 44% |
| Max | 55% |

| Quality analysis | | | |
|---|---|---|---|
| | Items | Values | Score |
| **1** | Signal quality | 0 or 2 | 0 |
| **2** | Area without IZ | 0 or 2 | 2 |
| **3** | Physiological signal propagation | 0 or 1 | 0 |
| **4** | Motor units identification | 0 or 1 | 0 |
| | Total | | 2 |

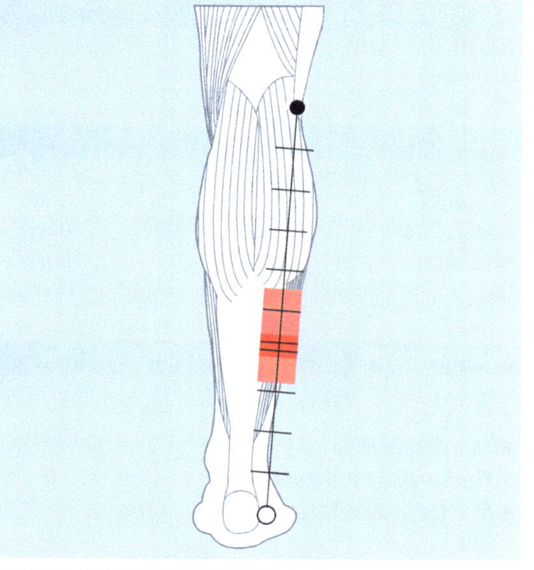

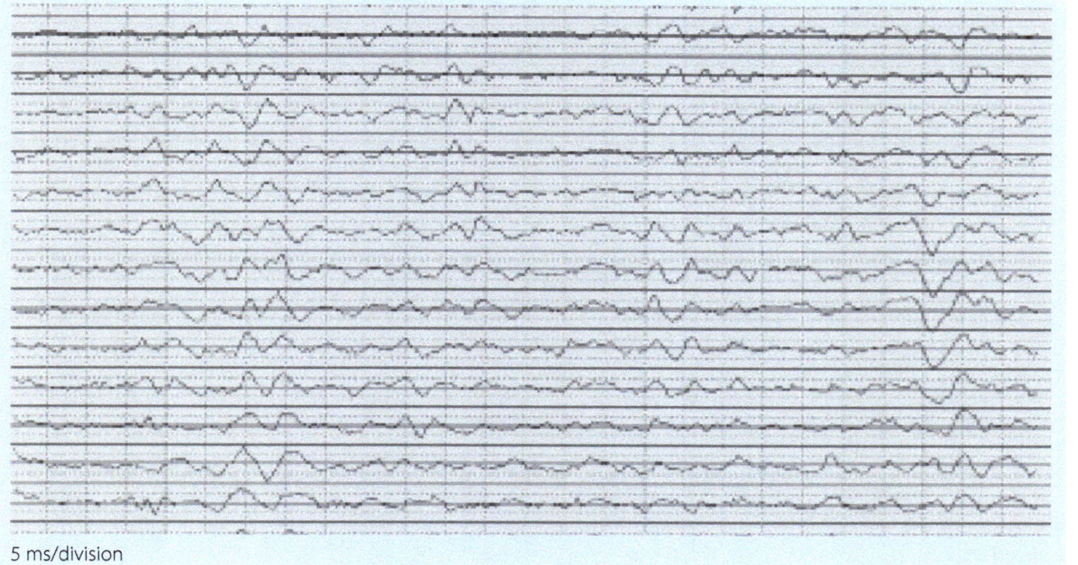

5 ms/division

## Tensor Fasciae Latae

- **Anatomical landmark frames (ALF)**: A line oriented 30° anterior to the reference line between the anterior superior iliac spine and the greater trochanter.
- **Experimental set up**: The subject lay on his or her side. An isometric contraction was then performed during abduction of the hip flexed at 20° and rotated externally.
- **Optimal electrode site**: Between 0 and 64 mm on the ALF or 114 mm away from the ALF.

| Subjects investigated | IZs detected |
|---|---|
| 20 Males | 15 |
| 20 Females | 12 |

| Results | |
|---|---|
| Min | 64 mm |
| 1st quartile | 79 mm |
| Median | 91 mm |
| 3rd quartile | 98 mm |
| Max | 114 mm |

| Quality analysis | | |
|---|---|---|
| Items | Values | Score |
| **1** Signal quality | 0 or 2 | 2 |
| **2** Area without IZ | 0 or 2 | 2 |
| **3** Physiological signal propagation | 0 or 1 | 0 |
| **4** Motor units identification | 0 or 1 | 1 |
| Total | | 5 |

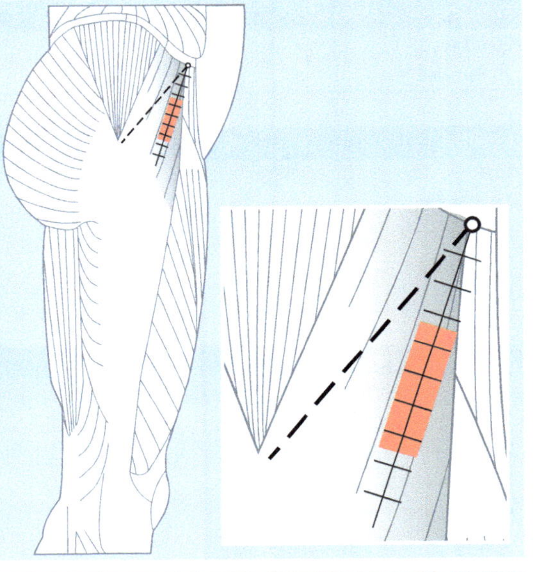

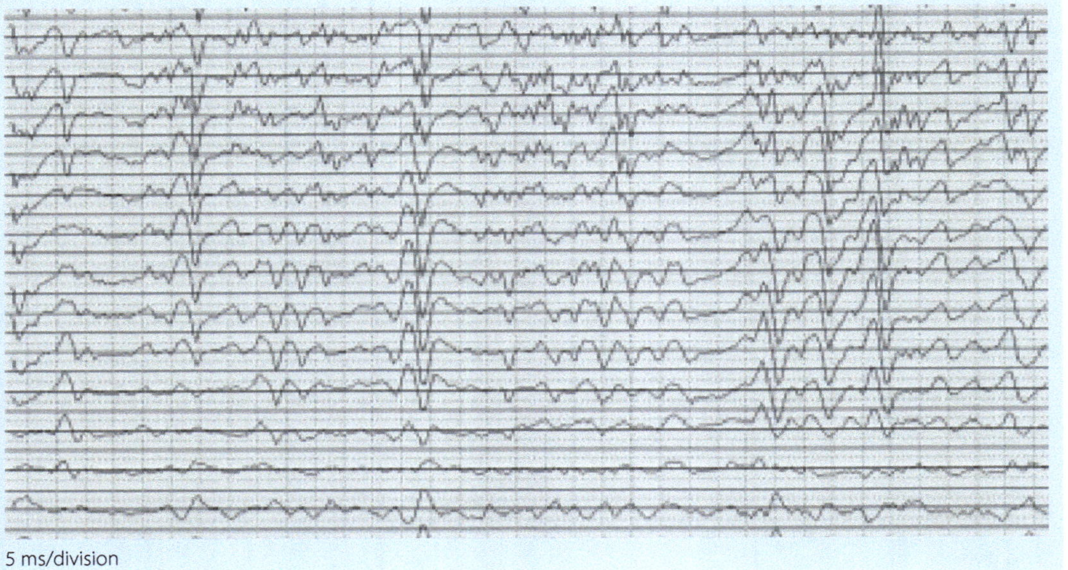

# Vastus Medialis

- **Anatomical landmark frames (ALF)**: A line on the distal portion of the muscle belly and oriented 50° with respect to the reference line between the medial side of the patella and the anterior superior iliac spine.
- **Experimental set up**: The subject was seated at the edge of the table. He or she then performed an isometric contraction during an extension of knee with the shank at 45° (0° = full extension).
- **Optimal electrode site**: Between 0 and 38 mm on the ALF or 88 mm away from the ALF.

| Subjects investigated | IZs detected |
|---|---|
| 20 Males | 20 |
| 20 Females | 20 |

| Results | |
|---|---|
| Min | 38 mm |
| 1st quartile | 53 mm |
| Median | 63 mm |
| 3rd quartile | 68 mm |
| Max | 88 mm |

| Quality analysis | | | |
|---|---|---|---|
| | Items | Values | Score |
| 1 | Signal quality | 0 or 2 | 2 |
| 2 | Area without IZ | 0 or 2 | 2 |
| 3 | Physiological signal propagation | 0 or 1 | 1 |
| 4 | Motor units identification | 0 or 1 | 1 |
| | Total | | 6 |

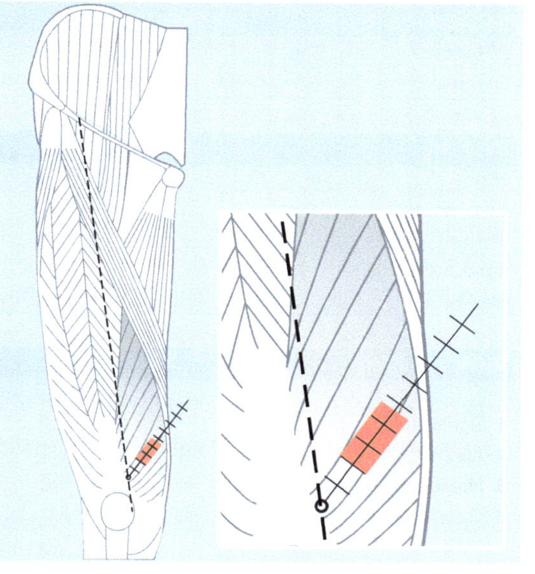

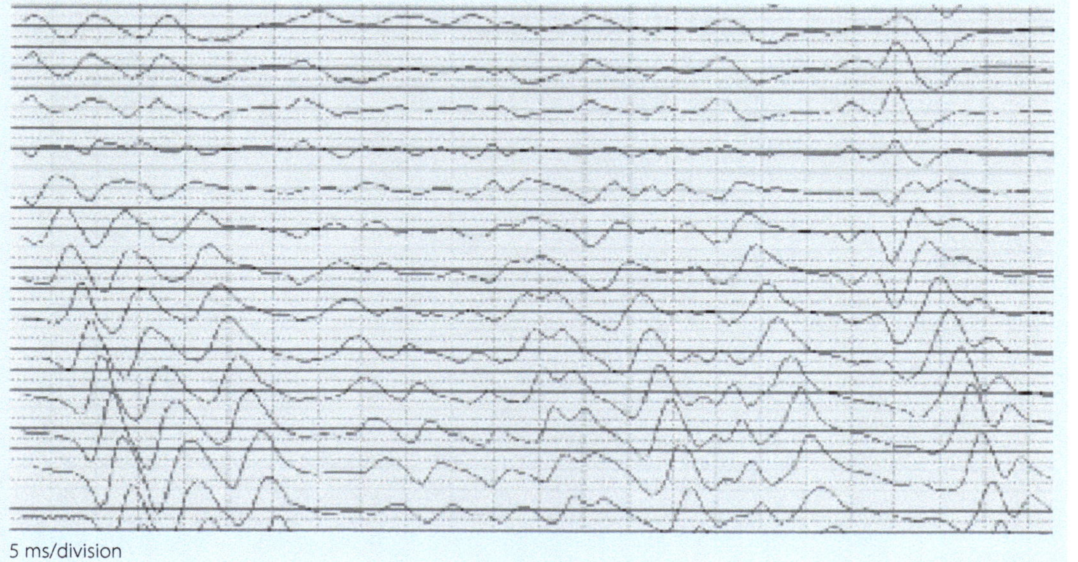

5 ms/division

## Rectus Femoris

- **Anatomical landmark frames (ALF)**: A line between the superior side of the patella and the anterior superior iliac spine.
- **Experimental set up**: The subject was seated at the edge of the table. He or she then performed an isometric contraction during an 80° extension of the knee (0° = full extension).
- **Optimal electrode site**: Between 0% and 50% or between 83% and 100% of the ALF.
- **Notes**: All 40 subjects showed clear motor unit action potentials propagation. Nine subjects showed multiple IZs.

| Subjects investigated | IZs detected |
|---|---|
| 20 Males | 12 |
| 20 Females | 14 |

| Results | |
|---|---|
| Min | 50% |
| 1st quartile | 56% |
| Median | 70% |
| 3rd quartile | 74% |
| Max | 83% |

| Quality analysis | | | |
|---|---|---|---|
| | Items | Values | Score |
| **1** | Signal quality | 0 or 2 | 0 |
| **2** | Area without IZ | 0 or 2 | 2 |
| **3** | Physiological signal propagation | 0 or 1 | 0 |
| **4** | Motor units identification | 0 or 1 | 1 |
| | Total | | 3 |

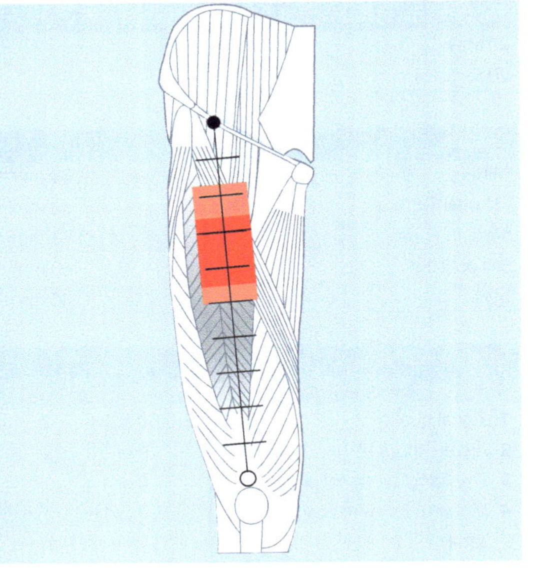

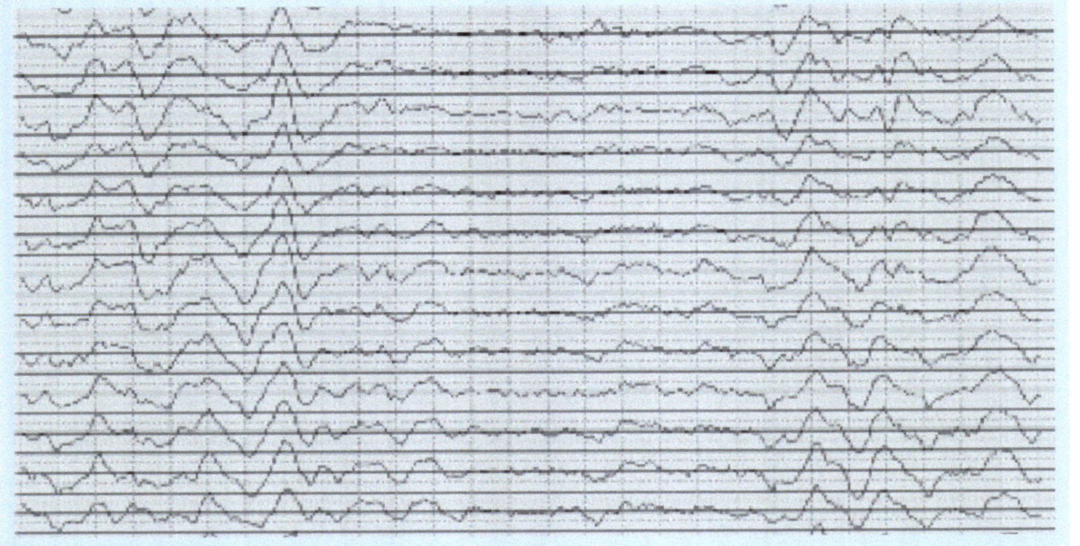

5 ms/division

# Vastus Lateralis

- **Anatomical landmark frames (ALF)**: A line on the distal portion of the muscle belly and oriented 20° with respect to the reference line between the lateral side of the patella and the anterior superior iliac spine.
- **Experimental set up**: The subject was seated at the edge of the table. He or she then performed an isometric contraction during an extension of knee with the shank at 80° (0° = full extension).
- **Optimal electrode site**: Between 0 and 43 mm on the ALF or 165 mm away from the ALF.

| Subjects investigated | IZs detected |
|---|---|
| 20 Males | 20 |
| 20 Females | 19 |

| Results | |
|---|---|
| Min | 43 mm |
| 1st quartile | 64 mm |
| Median | 83 mm |
| 3rd quartile | 106 mm |
| Max | 165 mm |

| Quality analysis | | |
|---|---|---|
| Items | Values | Score |
| **1** Signal quality | 0 or 2 | 2 |
| **2** Area without IZ | 0 or 2 | 2 |
| **3** Physiological signal propagation | 0 or 1 | 1 |
| **4** Motor units identification | 0 or 1 | 1 |
| Total | | 6 |

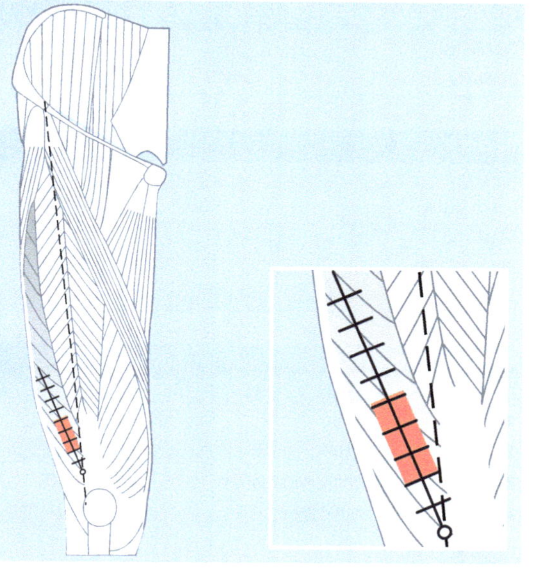

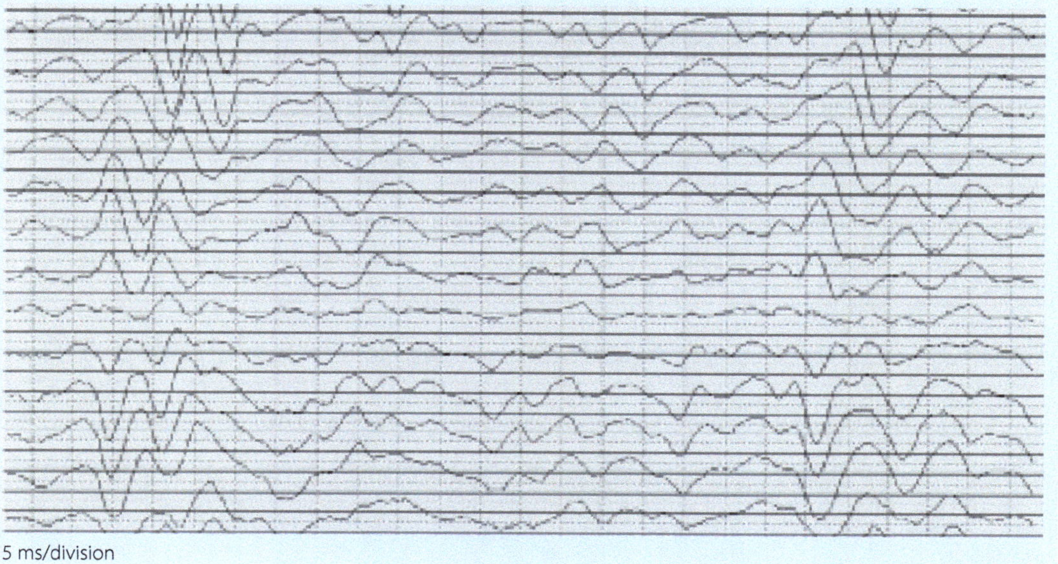

5 ms/division

# Tibialis Anterior

- **Anatomical landmark frames (ALF)**: A line between the tibial tuberosity and the intermalleolar line.
- **Experimental set up**: The subject was seated on a chair. An isometric contraction was then performed during a dorsal extension of the ankle.
- **Optimal electrode site**: Between 0% and 19% or between 51% and 100% of the ALF.
- **Notes**: In case of distal positioning of the electrode, the muscle belly is located proximally.

| Subjects investigated | IZs detected |
|---|---|
| 20 Males | 16 |
| 20 Females | 14 |

| Results | |
|---|---|
| Min | 19% |
| 1st quartile | 30% |
| Median | 34% |
| 3rd quartile | 38% |
| Max | 51% |

| Quality analysis | | | |
|---|---|---|---|
| | Items | Values | Score |
| 1 | Signal quality | 0 or 2 | 2 |
| 2 | Area without IZ | 0 or 2 | 2 |
| 3 | Physiological signal propagation | 0 or 1 | 0 |
| 4 | Motor units identification | 0 or 1 | 1 |
| | Total | | 5 |

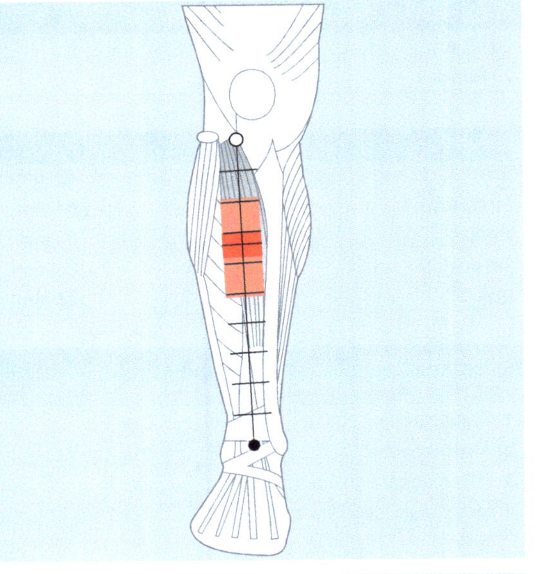

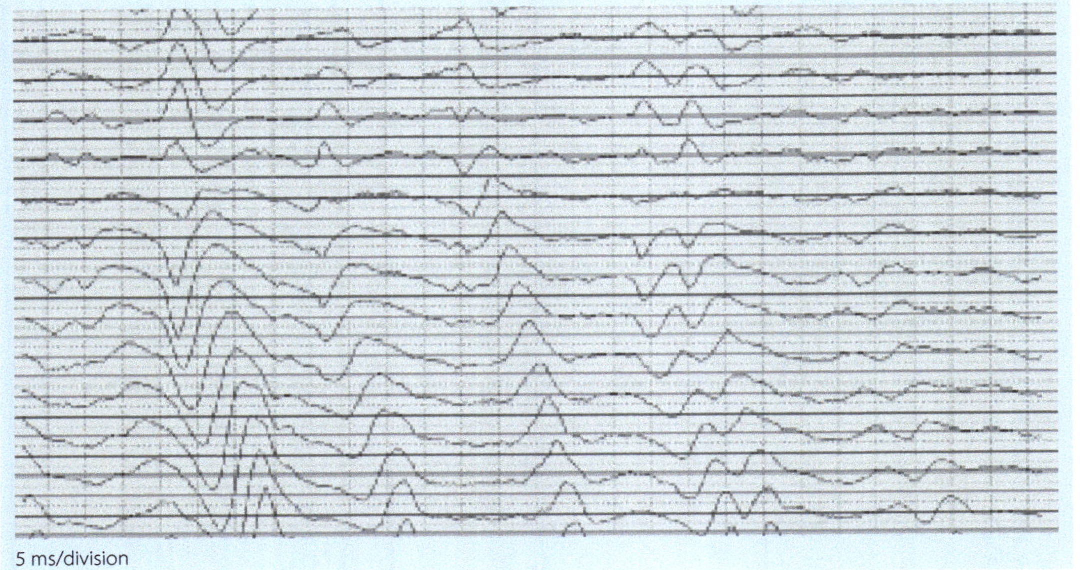

5 ms/division

## Peroneus Longus

- **Anatomical landmark frames (ALF)**: A line between the head of the fibula and the lateral malleolus.
- **Experimental set up**: The subject lay on his or her side. An isometric contraction was then performed during eversion of the foot.
- **Optimal electrode site**: After 38% of the ALF.
- **Notes**: In case of distal positioning of the electrode, the muscle belly is located proximally.

| Subjects investigated | IZs detected |
|---|---|
| 20 Males | 17 |
| 20 Females | 14 |

| Results | |
|---|---|
| Min | 5% |
| 1st quartile | 16% |
| Median | 20% |
| 3rd quartile | 32% |
| Max | 38% |

| Quality analysis | | | |
|---|---|---|---|
| | Items | Values | Score |
| **1** | Signal quality | 0 or 2 | 2 |
| **2** | Area without IZ | 0 or 2 | 2 |
| **3** | Physiological signal propagation | 0 or 1 | 0 |
| **4** | Motor units identification | 0 or 1 | 1 |
| | Total | | 5 |

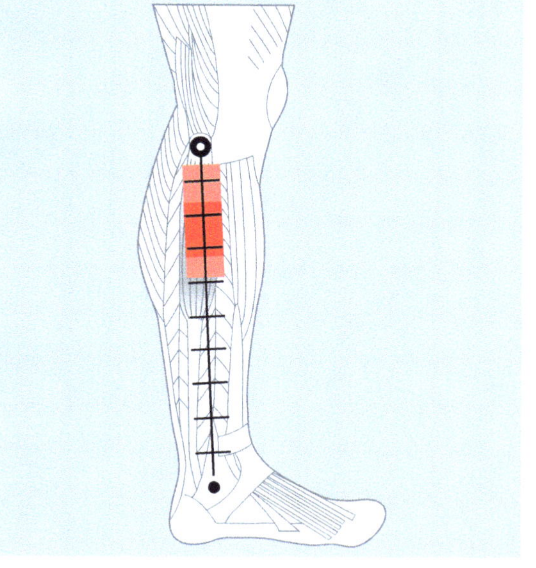

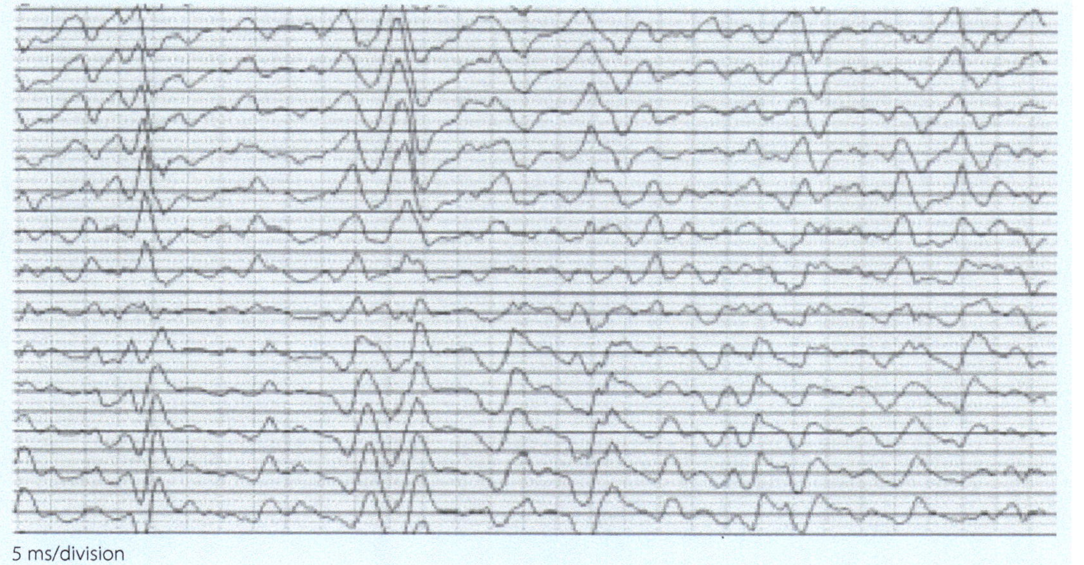

5 ms/division

# Additional Reading: Textbooks, Journals, and Special Journal Issues


**Textbooks and Proceedings of Congresses**

Basmajan J, De Luca CJ (1985) Muscles Alive. Williams and Wilkins, New York

Selected topics in surface electromyography for use in the occupational setting: expert perspectives (SuDoc HE 20.7102:SU 7) by U.S. Dept of Health and Human Services, 1992

Kumar S, Mital A (1996) Electromyography in Ergonomics. Taylor & Francis

Kasman GS, Cram JR, Wolf SL, Barton L (1997) Clinical applications in surface electromyography: chronic musculoskeletal pain. Aspen Publication

Cram J, Kasman G, Holtz J (1998) Introduction to surface electromyography. Aspen Publishers Inc., Gaithersburg, Maryland

Hermens HJ, Freriks B, Merletti R, Stegeman D, Blok J, Rau G, Disselhorst-Klug C, Hägg G, Roessingh Research and Development (1999) European Recommendations for Surface Electromyography: results of the SENIAM project. The Netherlands

Copies available from: Dr. ir. H.J. Hermens, PO Box 310, 7500 AH Enschede, The Netherlands; fax. +31-53-434 08 49; e-mail: info@seniam.org, website of project SENIAM: www.seniam.org

Christensen H, Sjøgaard G (1999) Symposium on muscular disorders in computer users: mechanisms and models. National Institute of Occupational Health, Copenhagen

Benvenuti F, Søgaard K, Disselhorst-Klug C, Farina D, Hermens H, Kadefors R, Laübli T, Orizio C (2004) Proceedings of the International Symposium on Neuromuscular Assessment in the Elderly Worker. Cooperativa Libraria Università di Torino (CLUT), Politecnico di Torino, ISBN 88-7992-191-6

Hermens HJ, Freriks B, Merletti R, Stegeman D, Blok J, Rau G, Disselhorst-Klug C, Hägg G (2000) Raccomandazioni Europee per l'Elettromiografia di Superficie. Edizione italiana a cura di Merletti R, Cooperativa Libraria Università di Torino (CLUT). Politecnico di Torino, ISBN 88-7992-1525

Merletti R (ed) (2000) Elementi di elettromiografia di superficie. Cooperativa Libraria Università di Torino (CLUT), Politecnico di Torino, ISBN 88-7922-153-3

Sandsjö L, Kadefors R (2001) Symposium on muscle disorders in computer users: scientific basis and recommendations. National Insitute for Working life, Göteborg

Merletti R, Parker PA (ed) (2004) Electromyography: physiology, engineering, and non invasive applications. IEEE Press and John Wiley & Sons

Weiss L, Silver J, Weiss J (2004) Easy EMG. Elsevier

Kamen G, Gabriel DA (2010) Essentials of Electromyography. Human Kinetics

**Journals**

Journal of Electromyography and Kinesiology. Elsevier; www.elsevier.com/locate/jelekin

Electroencephalogr Clin Neurophysiol Electromyogr Mot Control. Published/hosted by Elsevier Science, ISSN: 0924-980X; http://journalseek.net

Gait and posture, Elsevier, ISSN: 0966-6362; www.gaitposture.com

**Special Issues of Journals on EMG**

Intelligent data analysis in electromyography and electroneurography. Special issue of Medical Engineering and Physics, vol. 21, n. 6/7, 1999; www.elsevier.com/locate/medengphy

Proceedings of the European Commission on Surface EMG for non invasive assessment of muscles, Special issue of Journal of Electromyography and Kinesiology, vol. 10, n. 5, 2000

Monitoring muscles in motion, IEEE Engineering in Medicine and Biology Magazine, vol. 20, n. 6, 2001

Special issue on "Motor control and mechanisms of muscle disorders in computer users", European Journal of Applied Physiology, vol. 83, n. 2-3, 2003

Special issue on "Muscle function and dysfunction in the spine", Journal of Electromyography and kinesiology, vol. 13, n. 4, 2003

Special section on "Neuromuscular assessment in the elderly worker", Medical and Biological Engineering and Computing, vol. 42, n. 4, 2004

Special section on "On ASymmetry In Sphincters (OASIS): The role of asymmetry of sphincter innervation in incontinence". Enck P (ed) Digestion, vol. 69, n. 2, 2004

Special issue on Neuromuscular assessment of the Elderly Worker (Project NEW) Sjøgaard G, Hermens H (ed) European Journal of Applied Physiology, vol. 96, n. 2, 2006

Advances in Surface Electromyography. Merletti R (ed) Critical Reviews in Biomedical Engineering, vol. 38, n. 4, 2010

Special session on the electrode-skin interface and optimal detection of bioelectric signals. Merletti R (ed) Physiological Measurement, vol. 31, n. 10, 2010

# Subject Index

MIX
Papier aus verantwortungsvollen Quellen
Paper from responsible sources
FSC® C105338

If you have any concerns about our products,
you can contact us on
**ProductSafety@springernature.com**

In case Publisher is established outside the EU,
the EU authorized representative is:
**Springer Nature Customer Service Center GmbH**
**Europaplatz 3, 69115 Heidelberg, Germany**

Printed by Libri Plureos GmbH
in Hamburg, Germany